COMPETENCY MANUAL FOR

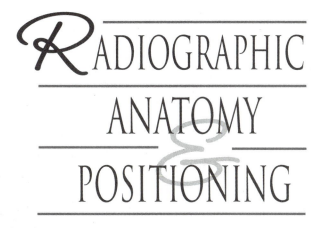

RADIOGRAPHIC ANATOMY & POSITIONING

Andrea Gauthier Cornuelle, MS, RT (R)
Associate Professor
Radiologic Technology
Department of Allied Health and Human Services, and Social Work
Northern Kentucky University
Highland Heights, Kentucky

APPLETON & LANGE
Stamford, Connecticut

Copyright © 1998 by Appleton & Lange
A Simon & Schuster Company

All rights reserved. This book, or any parts thereof, may not be used or reproduced in any manner without written permission. For information, address Appleton & Lange, Four Stamford Plaza, PO Box 120041, Stamford, Connecticut 06912-0041.

99 00 01 02/ 10 9 8 7 6 5 4 3 2

Prentice Hall International (UK) Limited, *London*
Prentice Hall of Australia Pty. Limited, *Sydney*
Prentice Hall Canada, Inc., *Toronto*
Prentice Hall Hispanoamericana, S.A., *Mexico*
Prentice Hall of India Private Limited, *New Delhi*
Prentice Hall of Japan, Inc., *Tokyo*
Simon & Schuster Asia Pte, Ltd., *Singapore*
Editora Prentice Hall do Brasil Ltda., *Rio de Janeiro*
Prentice Hall, *Upper Saddle River, New Jersey*

ISBN: 0–8385–8239–7

Acquisitions Editor: Kim Davies
Production Editor: Elizabeth Ryan
Designer: Janice Barsevich Bielawa

PRINTED IN THE UNITED STATES OF AMERICA

ISBN 0-8385-8239-7

90000

9 780838 582398

To the students who have used this manual
and offered suggestions for improvement, and
to my family for their never-ending support.

CONTENTS

PREFACE

This *Competency Manual* was developed to give simple step-by-step instructions for performing radiographic positioning. It was also designed as an evaluative tool for use in a laboratory or clinical setting. Various radiographic positioning texts were used as resources during the *Manual's* development. This *Manual* is not meant to be a comprehensive guide to all radiographic positioning. It includes descriptions of projections most commonly performed.

Each projection is divided into discrete tasks that must be performed for accurate patient positioning. Each **task analysis** has an introductory section that includes the projection name, student's objective, basic patient preparation, cassette type, film size, and orientation. The procedural portion of the task analysis includes special informational notes as well as identification of anatomy that should be demonstrated on the finished radiograph (Critical Anatomy) if the patient is correctly positioned. Space is included on each task analysis to indicate satisfactory and unsatisfactory performance when this manual is used for eval-

uation purposes. Drawings have been included with each task analysis to illustrate patient position, film placement, and central ray location. Although cassette sizes are stated in inches, metric conversions are included in chapter 1.

The *Competency Manual* can be used with or without the checklist to evaluate student performance. The *Manual* may also be used as a quick reference for the technologists and students or as a procedural manual within a department. Space is found at the end of each projection for notes.

A tremendous amount of time and energy have gone into the production of this *Manual*. As with any project of this magnitude, editing and revision are on-going processes. Constructive comments and suggestions would be accepted gratefully. The author hopes this *Manual* will be beneficial to the student and technologist, not only for instruction and evaluation, but also as a reference.

Andrea Gauthier Cornuelle

ACKNOWLEDGMENTS

In one form or another, this *Competency Manual* has been in existence for over 12 years. I owe special thanks to Carlos Soto, my first program director, who asked me to create a manual that could be used to document laboratory competence, and to Katherine C. Rosenthal for collaborating with me on the first edition. My colleague, Diane Gronefeld, graciously agreed to review content during the first major revision stage seven years ago and has continued to offer suggestions for improvement since that time.

I want to recognize and thank Kathy Stewart and Beth Merten for the many hours they spent developing the art for this manual. The work was time consuming as they toiled to produce drawings that accurately illustrate each patient position.

Last, my family deserves more thanks than I can possibly express. They have been patient and supportive throughout the entire process.

A.G.C.

INTRODUCTION TO RADIOGRAPHIC POSITIONING

This manual was developed to provide students and practicing radiographers with step-by-step guidelines necessary to position patients accurately for radiographic examinations. When following these guidelines, however, it is important to remember that they are just that—guidelines. There is often more than one way to achieve the desired outcome. No single guideline can apply to all patients in all situations.

This manual should be used as a practical tool, but, as with all tools, the user must use common sense and think through all situations, deciding when it is necessary to vary from a standard guideline. For example, when centering a patient for a KUB (kidneys, ureters, and bladder) examination, the standard guideline is to center the central ray to the level of the iliac crests. With many male patients, however, the symphysis pubis and part of the bladder area would be missed if the central ray were not directed inferior to the iliac crests. On this same patient, the radiographer may have to center above the iliac crests to include the kidneys on the radiograph. In addition, positioning protocols vary from one department to another. The radiographer must follow protocol as stated in the department's policy and procedure manual. It is, therefore, important to always double-check your work and make adjustments in centering and positioning as necessary.

▶ PROCEDURAL CONSIDERATIONS

Patient Care

Communication with the patient is a vitally important part of the radiographer's job. Because radiographic examinations are usually fairly brief, the radiographer must quickly establish a good rapport with the patient. Most often, the first contact the radiographer has with the patient is in the waiting room when the patient's name is called. After the radiographer correctly identifies the patient, the patient may be instructed to enter a dressing booth to change into a patient gown. Instructions should be thorough and clear. It is also important to remember that the patient may be feeling a loss of privacy and feel somewhat embarrassed by the new attire, especially if it is too short, too small, or open in the back. Help the patient feel comfortable.

A thorough patient history relevant to the requested examination is important for all radiographic examinations. This information should be conveyed to the radiologist who will interpret the films. Patient histories should be specific. Stating that the patient is experiencing pain at the base of the 5th metatarsal could change an interpretation from "probably normal" to "possible fracture" when the radiologist sees something that could be a normal variant. Stating that the patient "fell" may not provide adequate information and could result in an inaccurate interpretation of the study.

The radiographer is also responsible for providing procedural information before, during, and after the examination. When the patient understands what is expected, he or she is more likely to cooperate fully, leading to better-quality radiographs.

Last, while the radiographer may remember few details about the patients or procedures performed in a given week, the patients *will* remember many details about the radiographer and the care received. Good impressions count!

Positioning Terminology

Projection is a term used to describe the direction of the central ray as it passes through the body. An *AP projection*, therefore, is one in which the central ray enters the anterior aspect of the body and exits at the posterior aspect. The term *position* is used to describe the actual position in which the patient is placed. To accurately position a patient for a radiographic projection, the radiographer must be familiar with various terms. Anatomical planes, directional terms, and positioning terms used throughout this text are summarized in Tables 1–1 to 1–3.

TABLE 1–1. Anatomical Planes

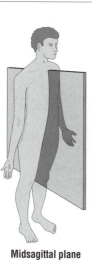

Midsagittal plane	Midcoronal (frontal) plane

Midaxillary Plane: A coronal plane that passes through the axilla at the junction of the arm and thorax when the arms are at a 90° angle with the body. Although this term is often used synonymously with midcoronal plane, they are not necessarily the same.

Sagittal Plane: Any plane dividing the body into right and left sides; the **midsagittal plane** divides the body into *equal* right and left sides.

Coronal Plane: Any plane dividing the body into anterior and posterior parts; the **midcoronal plane** divides the body into *equal* front and back parts.

From Cornuelle AG, Gronefeld DH. Radiographic Anatomy & Positioning: An Integrated Approach. *Stamford, Conn.: Appleton & Lange; 1998.*
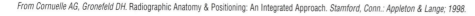

TABLE 1–2. Positioning Terminology

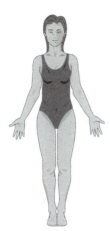

Anatomical position

Anatomical Position: The standing, erect position of the body with all anterior surfaces facing forward; the arms are down with palms forward.

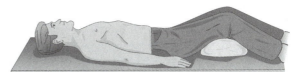

Supine (dorsal recumbent) position.

Supine: Lying flat on the back.

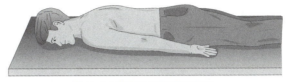

Prone (ventral recumbent) position.

Prone: Lying face down.

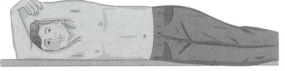

Right lateral recumbent position.

Lateral: Erect or recumbent position, 90° from true AP or PA.

Oblique: The patient is rotated between lateral and prone or supine position; the amount of obliquity may vary depending on the structure to be demonstrated.

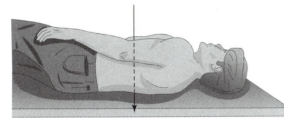

RPO (right posterior oblique) position; AP oblique projection.

Right Posterior Oblique Position: The right posterior side of the patient is nearest the film; the reverse of left anterior oblique.

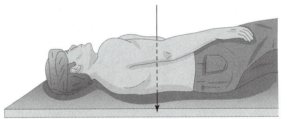

LPO (left posterior oblique) position; AP oblique projection.

Left Posterior Oblique Position: The left posterior side of the body is nearest the film; the reverse of right anterior oblique.

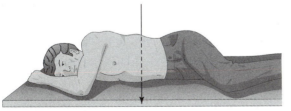

RAO (right anterior oblique) position; PA oblique projection.

Right Anterior Oblique Position: The right anterior side of the body is nearest the film; the reverse of left posterior oblique.

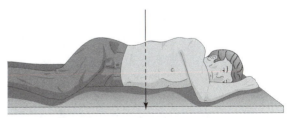

LAO (left anterior oblique) position; PA oblique projection.

Left Anterior Oblique Position: The left anterior side of the body is nearest the film; the reverse of right posterior oblique.

continued

TABLE 1–2. Positioning Terminology (continued)

Decubitus Position: The patient is recumbent; in radiography, usually implies the use of a horizontal beam; used to identify air–fluid levels or free air in a body cavity.

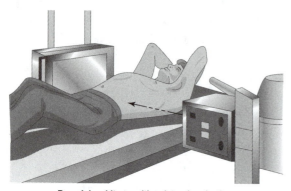

Dorsal decubitus position; lateral projection.

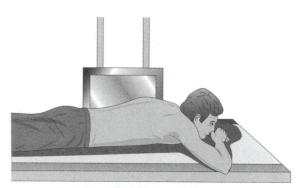

Ventral decubitus position; lateral projection.

Dorsal Decubitus: The patient is supine with the central ray passing horizontally from one side to the other.

Ventral Decubitus: The patient is prone with the central ray passing horizontally from one side to the other.

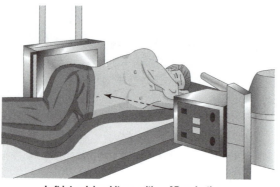

Left lateral decubitus position; AP projection.

Lateral Decubitus: The patient is lying on either the right or left side; the central ray travels horizontally either from front to back or back to front; when the patient is lying on the left side, it is termed a **left lateral decubitus.**

From Cornuelle AG, Gronefeld DH. Radiographic Anatomy & Positioning: An Integrated Approach. *Stamford, Conn.: Appleton & Lange; 1998.*

Film Sizes

Radiographic film and cassettes come in many different sizes to fit various needs. Not all radiology departments or offices will have all the sizes available. For this reason, more than one acceptable film or cassette size may be identified for many of the projections included in this manual.

Film and cassettes are currently measured in two different ways: inches and centimeters. Although the metric-sized film is not necessarily the same size as the standard unit film, they are often used interchangeably. For example, a 24 cm × 30 cm film is slightly smaller than a 10 in. × 12 in. film, but in departments that stock only 24 cm × 30 cm

film, this size is often referred to as 10 in. × 12 in. film. Because most radiographers use the standard unit sizes in practice, recommended film sizes in this manual will be in inches. Use the following chart to find the corresponding size in centimeters.

Standard Unit (inches)	Metric Unit (centimeters)
8 in. × 10 in.	20 cm × 25 cm
9 in. × 9 in.	24 cm × 24 cm
10 in. × 12 in	24 cm × 30 cm
11 in. × 14 in.	28 cm × 35 cm
7 in. × 17 in.	18 cm × 43 cm
14 in. × 17 in.	35 cm × 43 cm

TABLE 1–3. Directional/Relationship Terminology

Anterior

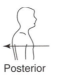

Posterior

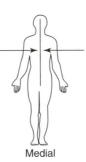

Medial

Lateral

Anterior/Ventral: The front or forward aspect of the body or body part.

Posterior/Dorsal: The back part of the body or body part.

Medial/Mesial: Toward the median plane or middle of a part; opposite of lateral (eg, the spine is medial to the kidneys).

Lateral: Away from the median plane or middle of a part; opposite of medial (eg, the kidneys are lateral to the spine).

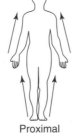

Distal

Proximal

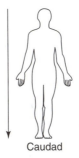

Caudad

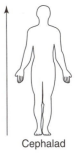

Cephalad

Distal: Parts furthest from the point of origin or attachment (eg, the fingers are distal to the wrist); opposite of proximal.

Proximal: Parts closest to the point of origin or attachment (eg, the elbow is proximal to the wrist); opposite of distal.

Caudad/Caudal/Inferior: Away from the head or toward the tail or feet; opposite of cephalad.

Cephalad/Cephalic/Cranial/ Superior: Pertaining to or toward the head; opposite of caudad.

From Cornuelle AG, Gronefeld DH. Radiographic Anatomy & Positioning: An Integrated Approach. *Stamford, Conn.: Appleton & Lange; 1998.*

Cassette Orientation

Most cassettes are rectangular in shape and may be positioned crosswise or lengthwise relative to the body part. Radiology departments and offices usually have specific guidelines pertaining to the orientation, or positioning, of the cassette. These policies may be due to physician preference or may be adapted to meet patient condition. The recommendations in this manual relative to cassette orientation may be changed to fit the department routine. Generally speaking:

1. The long side of the cassette should be parallel to the long axis of long bones or other long structures,
2. When two projections are going to be included on one film, the cassette is masked crosswise. An exception to this is the foot. Although both the AP and oblique foot projections are generally included on one film, the cas-

sette is masked lengthwise because the foot is a long structure.

Although there may be exceptions to these two rules, they should serve as a guide when orienting the cassette.

Using Lead Identification Markers

Lead markers are used to identify the right or left side of the patient, the patient's position, or a specific film in a series of films. They provide necessary information important in patient diagnosis. For medicolegal reasons, films should be correctly marked before processing. To avoid superimposition on critical anatomy and to assure inclusion in the collimated area, markers must be strategically placed on the cassette. Some radiology departments may have their own specific guidelines for marker use; however, the following general rules for using lead markers should be helpful in determining marker placement for each projection.

RULES FOR USING LEAD MARKERS

1. Right or left markers *must* be used on *all** films.
2. Markers should be placed on the cassette where they will be seen clearly on the radiograph, while not obscuring required anatomy.
   a. Markers should not be placed over the patient identification blocker.
   b. Markers should be placed within the collimation field.
   c. Markers should be placed away from an area where lead shielding on the patient or table may obscure the markers.
3. Markers must be placed appropriately to identify the *patient's* right or left side.
4. When radiographing the extremities and hip or shoulder girdles, markers should be placed on the lateral side of the body part.
5. When using one film for two projections of the same body part (eg, PA and oblique right hand), only one of the projections must be marked.
6. If bilateral projections (eg, right and left AP knees) are positioned on one film, both right and left markers should be used to identify the corresponding sides.
7. Auxiliary markers (eg, post-evac, post-void, minute markers, etc) should be used whenever possible and positioned away from the critical anatomy.
8. When performing lateral decubitus projections, a marker indicating the side that is up should be placed on the upside of the cassette, away from any anatomy of interest.
9. For lateral projections, a marker indicating the side closest to the film should be used.
10. When radiographing the spine in the lateral position, markers should be placed on the cassette anterior to the spine to be clearly visualized (not "burned out" or obscured by lead masking on the table behind the patient).
11. When radiographing the chest, abdomen, or spine in an oblique position, the side nearest the film is generally marked. For example, when obtaining an LPO projection of the lumbar spine, a left marker would be placed on the cassette to identify the patient's left side. When both sides are on the film (eg, barium enema or oblique chest), either marker can be used.**

*****Exception:** To prevent superimposition of the marker on critical anatomy, many hospitals have a policy restricting marker use in surgery.

****The marker may also be used to identify the anatomical structure(s) seen on the projection. For example, an LPO position is used to demonstrate the right sacroiliac joint; therefore, a right marker could be used. Radiographers should follow department policy when using markers.

From Cornuelle AG, Gronefeld DH. Radiographic Anatomy & Positioning: An Integrated Approach. *Stamford, Conn.: Appleton & Lange; 1998.*

Radiation Protection

One of the primary responsibilities of the radiographer is to protect others from unnecessary exposure to ionizing radiation. Two methods the technologist can use to minimize patient dose are cited throughout this text—collimation and gonadal shielding. Although gonadal shielding may not be necessary for all anatomical areas and for all patients (ie, elderly patients), it is a habit the radiographer should adopt. Those who shield patients on a regular basis never have to stop to consider whether a female patient may be pregnant or what potential effects the radiation may have on the patient.

Closure

Patient positioning may seem awkward and tedious at first; however, the student radiographer will soon feel comfortable performing radiographic examinations. If knowledge of basic patient positioning is acquired for agile, cooperative patients, the radiographer can quickly learn to adapt basic positioning for those patients who are unable to assume the textbook position.

RESPIRATORY SYSTEM

- ► PA CHEST
- ► LATERAL CHEST
- ► PA OBLIQUE CHEST (RAO & LAO)
- ► LATERAL DECUBITUS (AP OR PA) CHEST
- ► LORDOTIC CHEST (LINDBLOOM METHOD)

▶ PA CHEST

OBJECTIVE: After practice, each student will position a patient for a PA projection of the chest.

PATIENT PREP: Remove all clothing and jewelry from the waist up; gown patient.

FILM: 14 in. × 17 in. lengthwise or crosswise, grid or non-grid.

TASK ANALYSIS		CORRECTLY PERFORMED?	
MAJOR STEPS	KEY INFORMATION	YES	NO
1. Assist the patient to an erect position facing the upright grid device or cassette holder.	If the patient is unable to sit or stand, an AP projection may be obtained with the patient sitting or lying supine; a horizontal beam is required to demonstrate air–fluid levels.		
2. Center the midsagittal plane of the body to the midline of the film with the patient's weight equally distributed on both feet.			
3. Adjust the height of the cassette so the upper border of the film is 1 1/2 to 2 in. above the top of the shoulders.	Women with large pendulous breasts should be asked to pull them superiorly and laterally.		
4. Extend the chin upward so it rests on the top of the cassette holder, if possible; adjust the head so there is no rotation.	The chin should be "stretched up" somewhat. When using an upright grid device, it may be impossible to extend the chin over the top edge.		
5. Position the patient with the backs of the hands on the hips; depress the shoulders and roll them forward to contact the cassette holder.	Make sure the hands are not high enough to be in the lung fields. The shoulders should be relaxed. Immobilize unsteady patients with a restraining band.		
6. Using 72-in. SID, direct the central ray to the midline of the patient at the level of T-7.	T-7 lies approximately 7 to 8 in. below the spinous process of C-7; the central ray will enter near the level of the inferior angles of the scapulae. The central ray may not be centered to the cassette.		
7. Collimate to include the apices, lateral margins of the ribs, and costophrenic angles; use gonadal shielding.	The upper airway should also be included in small children.		
8. Make the exposure during suspended *inspiration,* after the 2nd deep breath.	To demonstrate pneumothorax, foreign body, and fixation of the diaphragm, an additional full expiration radiograph may be needed.		

CRITICAL ANATOMY: Heart shadow, aortic arch, both lungs, hilum, apices, costophrenic angles, the air-filled trachea, and both hemidiaphragms.

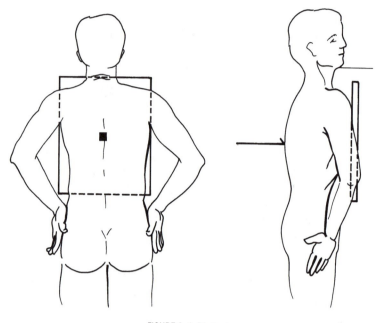

FIGURE 2–1. PA chest.

NOTES
....

► LATERAL CHEST

OBJECTIVE: After practice, each student will position a patient for a lateral projection of the chest.

PATIENT PREP: Remove all clothing and jewelry from the waist up; gown patient.

FILM: 14 in. × 17 in. lengthwise, grid or non-grid.

TASK ANALYSIS		CORRECTLY PERFORMED?	
MAJOR STEPS	KEY INFORMATION	YES	NO

1. Assist the patient to a lateral erect position next to the upright grid device or cassette holder: a. A left lateral position is used to demonstrate the heart and left lung. b. The right lateral position demonstrates the right lung.	The lateral projection obtained may depend on the department routine or pathology; a left lateral projection is usually preferred. The patient's feet should be separated slightly with weight equally distributed.		
2. Adjust the height of the cassette so the upper border of the film is 1 1/2 to 2 in. above the top of the shoulders.	The height of the cassette should remain approximately the same as for the PA projection.		
3. Extend the arms directly upward, flex the elbows, and, with forearms resting on head, grasp the elbows with the opposite hands to hold the arms in position.	Demonstrating this position while standing in front of the patient will help. An unsteady patient may grasp an IV stand or other device for support.		
4. With the patient standing up straight, center the thorax to the cassette.	The midcoronal plane should be centered to the midline of the film. Do not have the patient lean in against the cassette or lean forward or backward.		
5. Using 72-in. SID, direct the central ray to the midline of the patient at the level of T-7.	T-7 lies approximately 3 to 4 in. inferior to the manubrial notch. The central ray may not be centered to the cassette.		
6. Recheck to make sure the patient is not rotated or leaning.			
7. Collimate to include the lungs, spine, sternum, and costophrenic angles; use gonadal shielding.	Physicians may also want the upper airway included in small children.		
8. Make exposure during suspended *inspiration*, after the 2nd deep breath.			

CRITICAL ANATOMY: Heart shadow, aortic arch, posterior lungs, and retrosternal space.

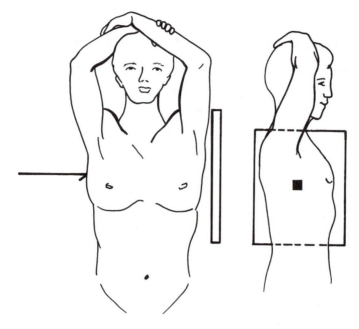

FIGURE 2–2. Lateral chest.

NOTES

▶ PA OBLIQUE CHEST (RAO & LAO)

OBJECTIVE: After practice, each student will position a patient for PA oblique projections of the chest.

PATIENT PREP: Remove all clothing and jewelry from the waist up; gown patient.

FILM: 14 in. × 17 in. lengthwise or crosswise, grid recommended.

TASK ANALYSIS		CORRECTLY PERFORMED?	
MAJOR STEPS	KEY INFORMATION	YES	NO
1. Assist the patient to an erect position facing the upright wall unit.			
2. Adjust the height of the wall unit so the upper border of the cassette is about 1 1/2 to 2 in. above the top of the shoulders.			
3. Rotate the patient so the midsagittal plane is at a 45° angle with the film plane.	The patient may be rotated 55° to 60° for the LAO in order to separate the heart and vertebral column. The patient's weight should be evenly distributed on both feet and the feet pointed in the direction the body is facing.		
4. Raise the arm furthest from the film to shoulder level with the hand resting on the wall unit.			
5. Flex the arm nearest the film and place the back of the hand on the hip.	Both arms should be clear of the lung fields.		
6. Adjust the shoulders to lie in the same transverse plane.			
7. With the patient standing up straight, center the thorax to the cassette.			
8. Using a 72-in. SID, direct the central ray perpendicular to the film plane at the level of T-7.	T-7 lies about 7 to 8 in. below the spinous process of C-7.		
9. Collimate to include the apices and thorax; use gonadal shielding.			
10. Make exposure during suspended *inspiration,* after the 2nd deep breath.			
11. Both oblique projections are performed.			

CRITICAL ANATOMY: *RAO*—Left lung, trachea, heart (especially left atrium), and right retrocardiac space. *LAO*—Right lung, trachea, heart.

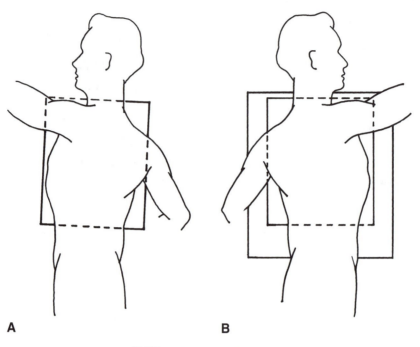

A   **B**

FIGURE 2–3. **A.** RAO chest. **B.** LAO chest.

NOTES
....

▶ LATERAL DECUBITUS (AP OR PA) CHEST

OBJECTIVE: After practice, each student will position a patient for a lateral decubitus (AP or PA) projection of the chest.

PATIENT PREP: Remove all clothing and jewelry from the waist up; gown patient.

FILM: 14 in. × 17 in. lengthwise with long axis of patient, grid or non-grid.

TASK ANALYSIS		CORRECTLY PERFORMED?	
MAJOR STEPS	KEY INFORMATION	YES	NO

1. Position the patient on the table or stretcher in the lateral recumbent position.

   The proper lateral projection will be requested.

   a. Fluid levels in the pleural cavity are best demonstrated with the patient lying on the affected side.

   The patient should lie in the lateral recumbent position for at least 10 minutes to allow fluid to settle or air to rise.

   b. Pneumothorax is best shown with the patient lying on the unaffected side.

2. To demonstrate a fluid level, elevate the side of interest several inches.

   The dependent side must be included on the film; use radiolucent sponges to elevate the body. Sponges are not needed if the patient is positioned on a stretcher in front of an upright table or wall unit.

3. Extend the arms above the head, keeping the upper shoulder directly over the dependent shoulder.

4. Adjust the thorax to a true lateral position.

   Stand at the head or foot of the table to check for rotation.

5. Place the cassette vertically against the anterior or posterior surface of the chest so the upper border is 2 in. above the top of the shoulders.

   An upright table or wall unit may also be used if the patient is positioned on a stretcher. If the patient is on the table, the cassette should be supported in a cassette holder or with sandbags.

6. Using 72-in. SID, direct the central ray horizontally to the level of T-7.

   If using a portable grid, the central ray should also be centered to the grid.

7. Collimate to include the apices, lateral margins of the ribs, and costophrenic angles; use gonadal shielding.

8. Make the exposure during suspended *inspiration,* after the 2nd deep breath.

CRITICAL ANATOMY: Lungs.

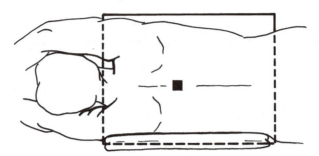

FIGURE 2–4. Left lateral decubitus chest.

NOTES
....

► LORDOTIC CHEST (LINDBLOOM METHOD)

OBJECTIVE: After practice, each student will position a patient for a lordotic projection of the chest using the Lindbloom method.

PATIENT PREP: Remove all clothing and jewelry from the waist up; gown patient.

FILM: 14 in. × 17 in. lengthwise or crosswise (entire chest); 11 in. × 14 in. crosswise (apices only).

TASK ANALYSIS		CORRECTLY PERFORMED?	
MAJOR STEPS	KEY INFORMATION	YES	NO
1. Position patient standing in front of, and about 1 ft away from, the upright cassette holder or grid device.	The patient should be facing the radiographic tube.		
2. Center the midsagittal plane to the midline of cassette.			
3. Place the backs of the patient's hands on the hips and roll the shoulders forward.			
4. Lean the patient backward in a position of extreme lordosis and rest the shoulders against the cassette.	This position may be uncomfortable for the patient.		
5. Using 72-in. SID, direct the central ray horizontally to the level of the midsternum.			
6. Center the cassette to the central ray.			
7. Collimate to include the apices, lateral margins of the ribs, and diaphragm; use gonadal shielding.	When using a smaller cassette, the diaphragm may not be included.		
8. Make the exposure during suspended *inspiration,* after the 2nd deep breath.			

NOTE: *If the patient cannot assume the lordotic position, assist the patient into the anatomical position (seated or standing) and direct the central ray 20° cephalad to a point approximately 2 in. lower than the midsternum and center the cassette to the central ray.*

CRITICAL ANATOMY: Apices.

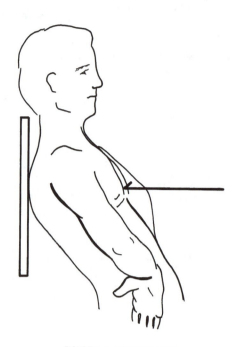

FIGURE 2–5. AP lordotic chest.

NOTES

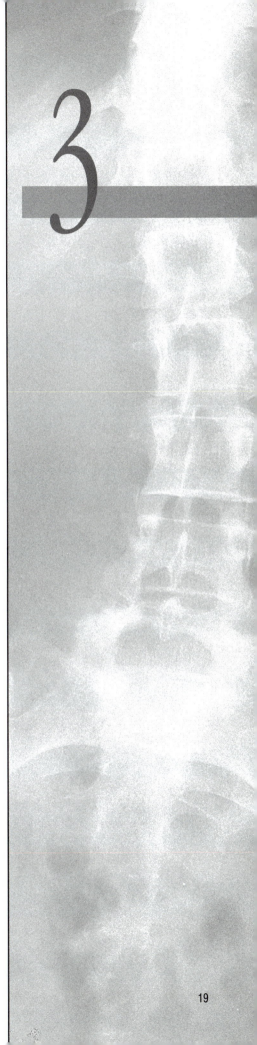

ABDOMEN

- ► AP ABDOMEN (KUB)
- ► UPRIGHT AP ABDOMEN
- ► LEFT LATERAL DECUBITUS ABDOMEN

▶ AP ABDOMEN (KUB)

OBJECTIVE: After practice, each student will position a patient for an AP projection of the abdomen in the supine position.

PATIENT PREP: Remove all clothing except socks and shoes; gown patient.

FILM: 14 in. × 17 in. lengthwise, grid required (large patients may require two films crosswise—one low and one high).

TASK ANALYSIS		CORRECTLY PERFORMED?	
MAJOR STEPS	KEY INFORMATION	YES	NO
1. Assist the patient to the supine position on the table.	A comparable projection can be obtained with the patient prone.		
2. Center the midsagittal plane to the midline of the table.	Align the patient to the long axis of the table. This can be checked by standing at the head or foot of the table.		
3. Position the patient's arms comfortably at the sides.			
4. Flex the knees and support with sandbags, sponges, or pillows.	Flexing the knees will move the back closer to the table top and will make the patient more comfortable.		
5. Direct the central ray perpendicular to the level of the iliac crests.	If the patient's abdomen is too large to be included on a 14 in. × 17 in. cassette lengthwise, two crosswise films may have to be taken. Make sure the symphysis pubis is included.		
6. Center the cassette to the central ray.			
7. Collimate to the abdomen and include the symphysis pubis; use gonadal shielding, if possible.			
8. Make the exposure during suspended *expiration.*			

CRITICAL ANATOMY: Renal shadows, psoas major muscles, and symphysis pubis.

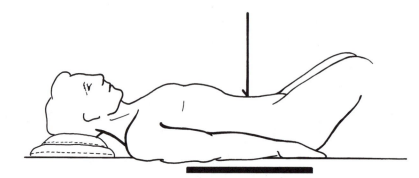

FIGURE 3–1. AP abdomen (KUB).

NOTES
....

► UPRIGHT AP ABDOMEN

OBJECTIVE: After practice, each student will position a patient for an upright AP projection of the abdomen.

PATIENT PREP: Remove all clothing (except socks and shoes) and necklaces; gown patient.

FILM: 14 in. × 17 in. lengthwise, grid required.

TASK ANALYSIS		CORRECTLY PERFORMED?	
MAJOR STEPS	KEY INFORMATION	YES	NO

1. Assist the patient to the erect position with the back against an upright grid device.	The patient may be standing or sitting.		
2. Center the midsagittal plane to the midline of the upright grid device.	A compression band may be used for immobilization.		
3. Position the patient's arms comfortably at the sides.			
4. Adjust the cassette so the upper edge is at the level of the axilla.	The center of the cassette will be approximately 2 to 3 in. above the iliac crests; this varies with the height of the patient. The diaphragm must be seen on the film to demonstrate any free air under the right hemidiaphragm.		
5. Direct the central ray perpendicular to the center of the cassette.			
6. Collimate to the abdomen; include the diaphragm.			
7. Make the exposure during suspended *expiration.*	The patient should be in the erect position for 10 to 20 minutes before the exposure is made.		

CRITICAL ANATOMY: Right hemidiaphragm and air–fluid levels within the intestines.

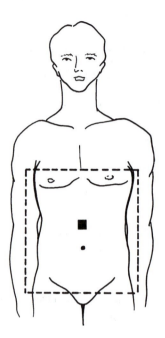

FIGURE 3–2. Upright abdomen.

NOTES
....

▶ LEFT LATERAL DECUBITUS ABDOMEN

OBJECTIVE: After practice, each student will position a patient in the left lateral decubitus position for the abdomen.

PATIENT PREP: Remove all clothing (except socks and shoes); gown patient.

FILM: 14 in. × 17 in. lengthwise, grid recommended.

TASK ANALYSIS		CORRECTLY PERFORMED?	
MAJOR STEPS	KEY INFORMATION	YES	NO

MAJOR STEPS	KEY INFORMATION	YES	NO
1. Assist the patient to the left lateral decubitus position on the table or stretcher.	The patient should lie in the lateral recumbent position for at least 10 minutes to allow any free air to accumulate under the right hemidiaphragm.		
2. Extend the arms above the head.	The right shoulder should be directly over the left shoulder.		
3. Bend the knees slightly.			
4. Adjust the thorax and pelvis to a true lateral position.	The right leg should be directly over the left leg. Stand at the head or foot of the table to check for rotation.		
5. Place the cassette vertically against the anterior or posterior surface of the abdomen *or* position the stretcher in front of the upright grid device.	Support the cassette with a cassette holder or sandbags. If using a grid cassette, make sure the central ray is centered to the grid to avoid grid cut-off.		
6. Position the cassette so the upper border is approximately level with the axilla and/or the center of the cassette is approximately 2 to 3 in. above the iliac crests.	The top edge of the cassette should be above the right lateral margin of the abdomen. The diaphragm must be included on the radiograph.		
7. Direct the central ray horizontally to the center of the cassette.			
8. Collimate to the abdomen; include the diaphragm.			
9. Make the exposure during suspended *expiration.*			

CRITICAL ANATOMY: Right hemidiaphragm and air–fluid levels within the intestines.

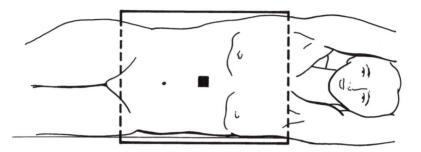

FIGURE 3–3. Left lateral decubitus abdomen.

NOTES
....

INTRODUCTION TO MUSCULOSKELETAL SYSTEM

Skeletal radiography includes examinations of upper and lower limbs, shoulder and pelvic girdles, vertebral column, skull, facial bones, and paranasal sinuses.

▶ POSITIONING CONSIDERATIONS

Although most radiography of the chest and abdomen is performed using the Bucky tray in the table or upright unit, many skeletal projections can be performed using a tabletop technique. To accomplish this, the part of interest is generally centered to the cassette first; the central ray is then centered to the part. Minor adjustment of the cassette centering can be made before making the exposure.

Although the primary objective is to place the part of interest in the middle of the film, there may be exceptions to this practice. When radiographing the ankle, for example, it is desirable to include as much of the lower leg as possible, especially in the case of traumatic injury. Typically the ankle joint would be centered to the film. To include more of the lower leg, however, the ankle can be positioned off-center lengthwise with the cassette. Although the joint is off-center to the cassette, the central ray should still be centered to the ankle joint.

In addition to the positioning terminology included in Chapter 1, Table 4–1 includes other terms related to skeletal radiography. To localize specific

TABLE 4–1. Part/Body Movement

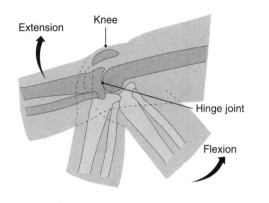

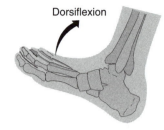

Dorsiflexion: Flexion between the lower leg and foot so the angle between the two structures is less than or equal to 90°.

Extension: Increasing the angle of a joint; straightening of a joint; the opposite of flexion; **hyperextension** refers to extension beyond normal limits.

Flexion: A decrease in the angle of a joint by bending; the opposite of extension; **hyperflexion** refers to over-flexion.

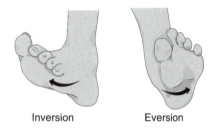

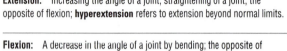

Inversion: Turning the foot inward at the ankle joint; the opposite of eversion.

Eversion: Turning the foot outward at the ankle joint; the opposite of inversion.

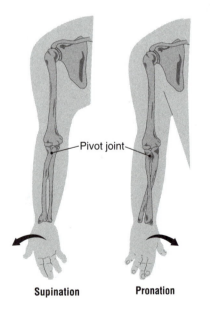

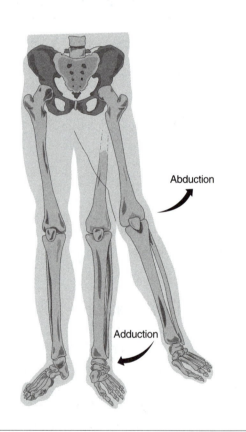

Adduction: Movement toward the midline of the body or body part; the opposite of abduction.

Abduction: Movement away from the midline of the body or body part; the opposite of adduction.

Supination: The act of turning onto one's back or turning the hand so the palm is facing upward; the opposite of pronation.

Pronation: The act of turning onto one's stomach or turning the hand so the palm is down; the opposite of supination.

continued

TABLE 4–1. Part/Body Movement (continued)

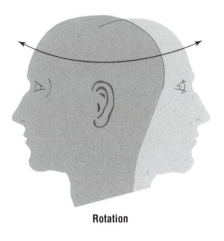

Rotation

Tilt

Rotation: Circular movement around a specified axis; eg, rotating the head from side to side.

Tilt: Moving the body part so the sagittal plane is not parallel with the long axis of the rest of the body and/or the table; used primarily to describe skull positioning, but may also describe alignment of the body or body part with the long axis of the film.

From Cornuelle AG, Gronefeld DH. Radiographic Anatomy & Positioning: An Integrated Approach. *Stamford, Conn.: Appleton & Lange; 1998.*

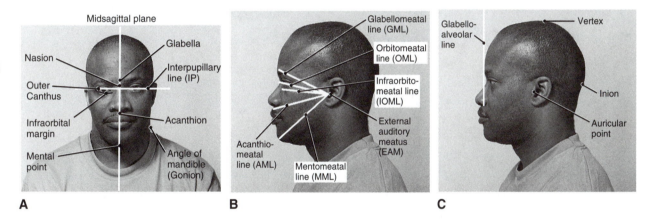

FIGURE 4–1. Topographical landmarks and positioning lines. **A.** Frontal perspective. **B** and **C.** Lateral perspective.

TABLE 4–2. Localization of Vertebrae

Bony Landmark	Corresponding Vertebrae
External acoustic meatus	1 in. superior to level of C-1
Mastoid tip	C-1
Gonion	C-3
Thyroid cartilage	C-5 (ranges from C4–6)
Vertebra prominens	C-7
Jugular notch	T2–3
1.5 in. superior to jugular notch	T-1
3–4 in. inferior to jugular notch	T-7
Sternal angle	T4–5
Xiphoid process	T-10
Lower costal margin	L2–3
Iliac crest	L4–5
Anterior superior iliac spine (ASIS)	S-2
Symphysis pubis	Coccyx

vertebrae, various bony landmarks can be used. These landmarks are summarized in Table 4–2. To accurately position the patient's head for skull, facial bone, or paranasal sinus projections, knowledge of specific centering points and positioning lines is required. Figure 4–1 illustrates these centering points and positioning lines.

Closure

Radiographic positioning is an art. Taking time to ensure that positioning is accurate before making an exposure contributes to more accurate diagnosis and helps prevent repeat radiographs, thereby reducing patient exposure and examination time.

UPPER LIMB (EXTREMITY)

5

► PA, PA OBLIQUE, & LATERAL FINGERS (2ND–5TH DIGITS)

OBJECTIVE: After practice, each student will position a patient for PA, PA oblique, and lateral projections of the fingers (2nd through 5th digits).

PATIENT PREP: Remove all jewelry from the affected hand.

FILM: 8 in. × 10 in., 9 in. × 9 in., or 10 in. × 12 in. masked in thirds crosswise.

TASK ANALYSIS		CORRECTLY PERFORMED?	
MAJOR STEPS	KEY INFORMATION	YES	NO

1. Seat the patient at the end of the table with the affected side nearest the table.

2. Rest the patient's arm on the table with the elbow flexed 90°.

3. Place the affected finger on the unmasked third of the cassette.
   a. *PA:* Pronate the hand and separate the fingers slightly.
   b. *PA oblique:* Rotate the finger to a 45° angle with the film plane.

   (Key information:) The finger must be parallel to the film plane to prevent foreshortening of the image and to demonstrate the joint spaces; use a radiolucent support to immobilize the finger and hand.

   c. *Lateral:* Turn the hand to the lateral position with the affected finger extended and the other fingers flexed out of the way.

   (Key information:) To reduce object–image receptor distance, internally rotate the hand for the 2nd digit and externally rotate the hand for the 3rd through 5th digits.

4. Center the proximal interphalangeal joint to the unmasked third of the cassette.

5. Direct the central ray perpendicular to the film through the proximal interphalangeal joint.

6. Collimate to include the finger and distal third of the metacarpal; use gonadal shielding.

CRITICAL ANATOMY: Proximal, distal, and middle phalanges; proximal and distal interphalangeal joints; and metacarpophalangeal joints.

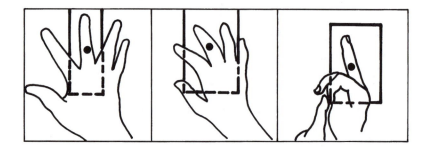

FIGURE 5–1. PA, oblique, and lateral 3rd finger.

NOTES

▶ AP, PA OBLIQUE, & LATERAL THUMB (1ST DIGIT)

OBJECTIVE: After practice, each student will position a patient for AP, PA oblique, and lateral projections of the thumb (1st digit).

PATIENT PREP: Remove all jewelry from the hand of the affected side.

FILM: 8 in. × 10 in., 9 in. × 9 in., or 10 in. × 12 in. masked in thirds crosswise.

TASK ANALYSIS		CORRECTLY PERFORMED?	
MAJOR STEPS	KEY INFORMATION	YES	NO

1. Seat the patient at the end of the table with the affected side nearest the table.

2. Rest the patient's arm on the table with the elbow flexed 90°.

3. Place the thumb on the unmasked third of the cassette.
   a. *PA oblique:* Pronate the hand and extend the fingers.
   b. *Lateral:* Arch the fingers and place the finger tips on the table; adjust so the thumb is in a true lateral position.
   c. *AP:* Internally rotate the hand to position the posterior surface of the thumb against the cassette.

When the hand is pronated, the thumb will naturally assume the oblique position.
Make sure the hand and fingers are not over the thumb.

This position may be somewhat difficult for the patient. Make sure the fifth finger is not over the thumb.

4. Center the metacarpophalangeal joint to the unmasked third of the cassette.

5. Direct the central ray perpendicular to the film through the metacarpophalangeal joint.

6. Collimate to include the thumb and carpometacarpal joint; use gonadal shielding.

CRITICAL ANATOMY: Proximal and distal phalanges, interphalangeal joint, metacarpophalangeal joint, and 1st carpometacarpal joint.

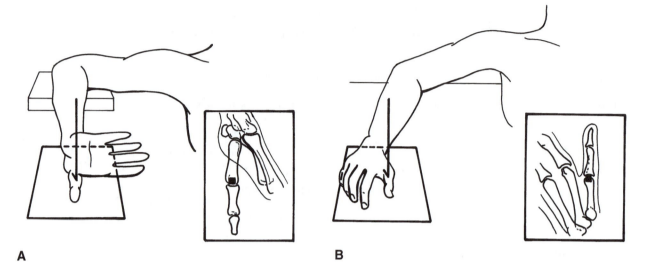

A   **B**

FIGURE 5–2. **A.** AP thumb. **B.** Lateral thumb.

NOTES

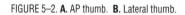

▶ PA HAND

OBJECTIVE: After practice, each student will position a patient for a PA projection of the hand.

PATIENT PREP: Remove all jewelry from the hand and wrist of the affected side.

FILM: 10 in. × 12 in. masked crosswise, or 8 in. × 10 in. lengthwise for single projection.

TASK ANALYSIS		CORRECTLY PERFORMED?	
MAJOR STEPS	KEY INFORMATION	YES	NO

1. Seat the patient at the end of the table with the affected side nearest the table.			
2. Rest the patient's arm on the table with the elbow flexed 90°.			
3. Pronate the hand on the unmasked half of the cassette.	Adjust the long axis of the hand and forearm parallel to the long axis of the unmasked half of the cassette; there should be no ulnar or radial flexion of the wrist.		
4. Center the 3rd metacarpophalangeal joint to the cassette.	When obtaining multiple projections on one film, position the part so that the projected images will be in alignment on the film.		
5. Spread the fingers slightly.	A small sandbag can be placed across the forearm to immobilize, if necessary.		
6. Direct the central ray perpendicular to the cassette through the third metacarpophalangeal joint.			
7. Collimate to include the hand, fingers, and at least 1 in. of the distal radius and ulna; use gonadal shielding.			

CRITICAL ANATOMY: Phalanges, interphalangeal joints, metacarpophalangeal joints, and metacarpals.

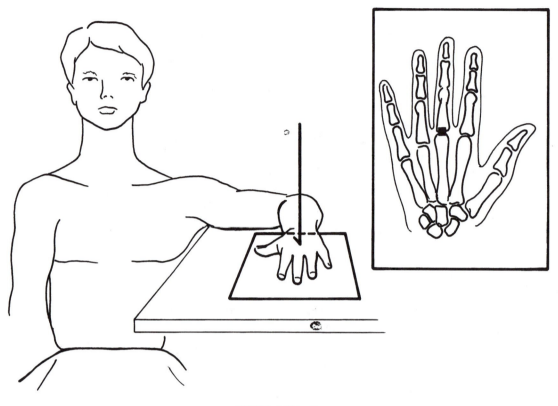

FIGURE 5–3. PA hand.

NOTES
....

▶ PA OBLIQUE HAND

OBJECTIVE:	After practice, each student will position a patient for a PA oblique projection of the hand.
PATIENT PREP:	Remove all jewelry from the hand and wrist of the affected side.
FILM:	10 in. × 12 in. masked crosswise, or 8 in. × 10 in. lengthwise for single projection.

TASK ANALYSIS		CORRECTLY PERFORMED?	
MAJOR STEPS	KEY INFORMATION	YES	NO
1. Seat the patient at the end of the table with the affected side nearest the table.			
2. Rest the patient's arm on the table with the elbow flexed 90°.			
3. Turn the patient's hand to the lateral position with the thumb side up and rest it on the unexposed half of the cassette.	This projection can be obtained on the same cassette as the PA projection, using lead masking.		
4. Rotate the hand medially with fingers extended.	When the fingers are the area of interest, they should be parallel to the film plane, if possible, to prevent foreshortening of the image. If no blood or body fluid is on the hand, a radiolucent support may be used for immobilization. When the fingers are not the area of interest, they may be flexed and allowed to rest on the cassette.		
5. Center the hand to the cassette.	A point midway between the 2nd and 3rd metacarpophalangeal joints should be centered to the cassette.		
6. Direct the central ray perpendicular to the cassette to a point halfway between the 2nd and 3rd metacarpophalangeal joints.			
7. Collimate to include the hand, fingers, and at least 1 in. of the distal radius and ulna; use gonadal shielding.			

CRITICAL ANATOMY: Phalanges, interphalangeal joints, metacarpophalangeal joints, metacarpals, and carpometacarpal joints (especially the 1st).

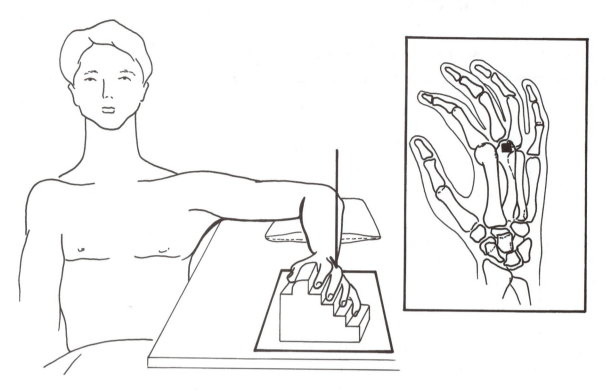

FIGURE 5–4. PA oblique hand.

NOTES
....

► LATERAL HAND IN EXTENSION

OBJECTIVE: After practice, each student will position a patient for a lateral projection of the hand.

PATIENT PREP: Remove all jewelry from the hand and wrist of the affected side.

FILM: 8 in. × 10 in. lengthwise or 10 in. × 12 in. masked crosswise.

TASK ANALYSIS		CORRECTLY PERFORMED?	
MAJOR STEPS	KEY INFORMATION	YES	NO
1. Seat the patient at the end of the table with the affected side nearest the table.			
2. Rest the patient's arm on the table with the elbow flexed 90°.			
3. Position the hand and forearm in the lateral position with the thumb extended in front of the palm.	The thumb should be fairly close to the palm without superimposition over the palm or fingers.		
4. Center the metacarpophalangeal joints to the cassette.			
5. Extend the fingers with the thumb parallel to the film plane; the thumb should be anterior to the carpals.	Some radiologists prefer the fingers to be flexed and separated to obtain a lateral view of each finger (fan lateral).		
6. Direct the central ray perpendicular to the cassette through the metacarpophalangeal joints.			
7. Collimate to include the hand, fingers, and at least 1 in. of the distal radius and ulna; use gonadal shielding.			

NOTE: *This projection is used routinely to localize foreign bodies and demonstrate anterior or posterior dislocation of fractures.*

CRITICAL ANATOMY: Superimposed metacarpals and superimposed 2nd through 5th digits.

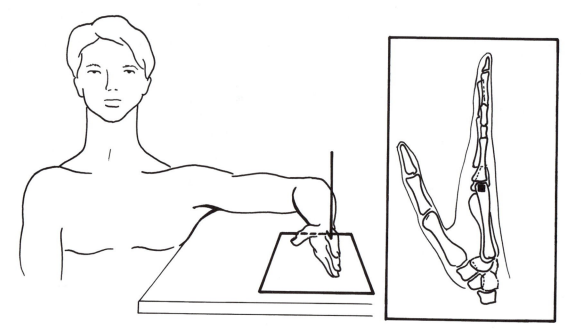

FIGURE 5–5. Lateral hand.

NOTES

EVALUATOR SIGNATURE _____ DATE _____

▶ PA WRIST

OBJECTIVE: After practice, each student will position a patient for a PA projection of the wrist.

PATIENT PREP: Remove all jewelry from the hand and wrist of the affected side.

FILM: 8 in. × 10 in., 9 in. × 9 in., or 10 in. × 12 in. masked crosswise.

TASK ANALYSIS		CORRECTLY PERFORMED?	
MAJOR STEPS	KEY INFORMATION	YES	NO

1. Seat the patient at the end of the table with the affected side nearest the table.			
2. Rest the patient's arm on the table with the elbow flexed 90°.	The patient should be seated low enough to allow the shoulder, elbow, and wrist to lie in the same horizontal plane; the upper arm should rest on the table.		
3. Pronate the hand on the unmasked half of the cassette.	Adjust the long axis of the hand and forearm so they are parallel to the unmasked half of the cassette; there should not be any radial or ulnar flexion.		
4. Center the midcarpal area to the unmasked section of the cassette.			
5. Arch the hand slightly.	Cupping the hand reduces the part-to-film distance. Place a radiolucent support under the fingers for immobilization, if necessary.		
6. Direct the central ray perpendicular to the cassette through the midcarpal area.			
7. Collimate to include at least 2 to 3 in. of the distal radius and ulna and one third of the proximal metacarpals; use gonadal shielding.			

CRITICAL ANATOMY: Scaphoid, lunate, capitate, distal trapezium, and hamate.

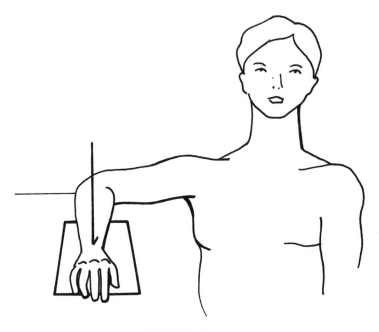

FIGURE 5–6. PA wrist.

NOTES
....

EVALUATOR SIGNATURE _____ DATE _____

▶ PA OBLIQUE WRIST (SEMIPRONATION)

OBJECTIVE: After practice, each student will position a patient for a PA oblique projection of the wrist.

PATIENT PREP: Remove all jewelry from the hand and wrist of the affected side.

FILM: 8 in. × 10 in., 9 in. × 9 in. or 10 in. × 12 in. masked crosswise.

TASK ANALYSIS		CORRECTLY PERFORMED?	
MAJOR STEPS	KEY INFORMATION	YES	NO

MAJOR STEPS	KEY INFORMATION
1. Seat the patient at the end of the table with the affected side nearest the table.	
2. Rest the patient's arm on the table with the elbow flexed 90° and the hand pronated.	The patient should be seated low enough to allow the shoulder, elbow and wrist to lie in the same horizontal plane; the upper arm should rest on the table.
3. Rotate the wrist and hand laterally to form a 45° angle with the cassette.	The 5th metacarpal will rest on the film. The use of a small 45°-angle sponge will immobilize the part and ensure duplication in follow-up films.
4. Center the midcarpal area to the unmasked section of the cassette.	
5. Direct the central ray perpendicular to the level of the navicular.	The central ray should enter approximately 1/2 in. distal to the radius.
6. Collimate to include at least 2 to 3 in. of the distal radius and ulna and one third of the proximal metacarpals; use gonadal shielding.	

CRITICAL ANATOMY: Scaphoid, trapezium, trapezoid, and 1st carpometacarpal joint.

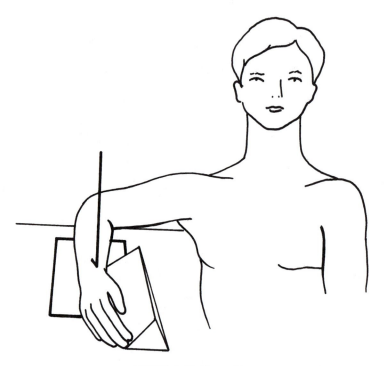

FIGURE 5–7. PA oblique wrist.

NOTES

EVALUATOR SIGNATURE _____ DATE _____

▶ AP OBLIQUE WRIST (SEMISUPINATION)

OBJECTIVE: After practice, each student will position a patient for an AP oblique projection of the wrist.

PATIENT PREP: Remove all jewelry from the hand and wrist of the affected side.

FILM: 8 in. × 10 in., 9 in. × 9 in., or 10 in. × 12 in. masked crosswise.

TASK ANALYSIS		CORRECTLY PERFORMED?	
MAJOR STEPS	KEY INFORMATION	YES	NO

1. Seat the patient at the end of the table with the affected side nearest the table.	The patient should be seated low enough to allow the shoulder, elbow, and wrist to lie in the same horizontal plane; the upper arm should rest on the table.		
2. Rest the patient's forearm on the table with the elbow extended and the hand supinated.			
3. Rotate the wrist and hand medially to form a 45° angle with the cassette.	The 5th metacarpal will rest on the cassette and the palm will be away from the film. The use of a small 45°-angle sponge will immobilize the part and ensure duplication in follow-up films.		
4. Center the midcarpal area to the unmasked section of the cassette.			
5. Direct the central ray perpendicular to the center of the midcarpal area.			
6. Collimate to include at least 2 to 3 in. of the distal radius and ulna and one third of the proximal metacarpals; use gonadal shielding.			

CRITICAL ANATOMY: Pisiform, triquetrum, and hamate.

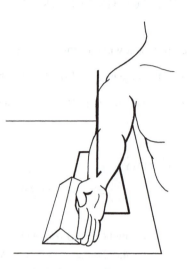

FIGURE 5–8. AP oblique wrist.

NOTES
....

EVALUATOR SIGNATURE _____ DATE _____

▶ LATERAL WRIST

OBJECTIVE: After practice, each student will position a patient for a lateral projection of the wrist.

PATIENT PREP: Remove all jewelry from the hand and wrist of the affected side.

FILM: 8 in. × 10 in., 9 in. × 9 in., or 10 in. × 12 in. masked crosswise.

TASK ANALYSIS		CORRECTLY PERFORMED?	
MAJOR STEPS	KEY INFORMATION	YES	NO

1. Seat the patient at the end of the table with the affected side nearest the table.			
2. Rest the patient's arm on the table with the elbow flexed 90°.	The patient should be seated low enough to allow the shoulder, elbow, and wrist to lie in the same horizontal plane; the upper arm should rest on the table.		
3. Place the wrist in the lateral position on the unmasked section of the cassette.			
4. Center the midcarpal area to the unmasked section of the cassette.			
5. Adjust the wrist and hand to a true lateral position.			
6. Direct the central ray perpendicular to the cassette through the midcarpal area.	The central ray should enter approximately 1/2 in. distal to the styloid process of the radius.		
7. Collimate to include at least 2 to 3 in. of the distal radius and ulna and one third of the proximal metacarpals; use gonadal shielding.			

CRITICAL ANATOMY: Trapezium, lunate, and pisiform.

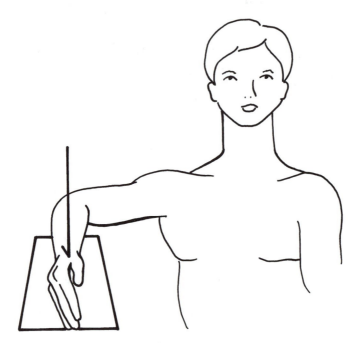

FIGURE 5–9. Lateral wrist.

NOTES
....

EVALUATOR SIGNATURE _____ DATE _____

▶ PA WRIST IN ULNAR & RADIAL FLEXION

OBJECTIVE: After practice, each student will position a patient for PA projections of the wrist in ulnar and radial flexion.

PATIENT PREP: Remove all jewelry from the hand and wrist of the affected side.

FILM: 8 in. × 10 in. or 9 in. × 9 in., masked crosswise for more than one projection.

TASK ANALYSIS		CORRECTLY PERFORMED?	
MAJOR STEPS	KEY INFORMATION	YES	NO
1. Seat the patient at the end of the table with the affected side nearest the table.	The patient should be seated low enough to allow the shoulder, elbow, and wrist to lie in the same horizontal plane.		
2. Set technical factors.	Because the position may be uncomfortable, technical factors should be set before positioning the wrist.		
3. Rest the patient's arm on the table with the elbow flexed 90°.			
4. Pronate the hand on the unmasked section of the cassette.	Adjust the long axis of the hand and forearm so they are parallel to the long axis of the unmasked section of the cassette.		
5. Center the midcarpal area to the cassette.			
6. *Ulnar flexion (radial deviation):* a. Deviate the hand outward in extreme ulnar flexion.	Hold the forearm in place while gently moving the hand outward to ulnar flexion. A sandbag can be used for immobilization, if necessary.		
b. Direct the central ray perpendicular to the cassette through the navicular.	To clearly delineate a fracture, the central ray must sometimes be angled 15° proximally or distally.		
7. *Radial flexion (ulnar deviation):* a. Deviate the hand inward to extreme radial flexion.	Hold the forearm in place while gently moving the hand inward to radial flexion. A sandbag can be used for immobilization, if necessary.		
b. Direct the central ray perpendicular to the cassette through the midcarpal area.			
8. Collimate to include the carpals and radiocarpal joint; use gonadal shielding.			

CRITICAL ANATOMY: *Ulnar flexion*—Scaphoid, lunate, trapezium, and trapezoid. *Radial flexion*—Hamate, pisiform, and triquetrum.

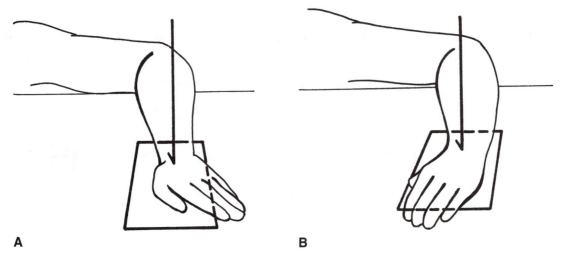

FIGURE 5–10. PA wrist in ulnar (**A**) and radial (**B**) flexion.

NOTES
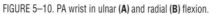

▶ TANGENTIAL CARPAL CANAL (GAYNOR–HART METHOD)

OBJECTIVE: After practice, each student will position a patient for a tangential projection of the carpal canal using the Gaynor–Hart method.

PATIENT PREP: Remove all jewelry from the hand and wrist of the affected side.

FILM: 8 in. × 10 in. lengthwise or 9 in. × 9 in.

TASK ANALYSIS		CORRECTLY PERFORMED?	
MAJOR STEPS	KEY INFORMATION	YES	NO
1. Seat the patient at the end of the table with the affected side nearest the table.	The patient should be seated low enough to allow the shoulder, elbow, and wrist to lie in the same horizontal plane.		
2. Set technical factors.	Because the position may be uncomfortable, technical factors should be set before positioning the wrist.		
3. Extend the elbow and rest the arm on the table, parallel to the table's long axis.	Because a central ray angle will be used, this step is very important for the reduction of unwanted distortion.		
4. Center the cassette to the level of the radial styloid process.			
5. With the hand pronated, hyperextend the wrist.	The long axis of the hand should be almost perpendicular to the cassette. Use the patient's opposite hand or other suitable device for immobilization.		
6. Direct the central ray at an angle of 25° to 30° to the long axis of the hand at a point 1 in. distal to the base of the 4th metacarpal.			
7. Collimate to include the carpals and metacarpals; use gonadal shielding.			

CRITICAL ANATOMY: Trapezium, pisiform, and hamular process of the hamate.

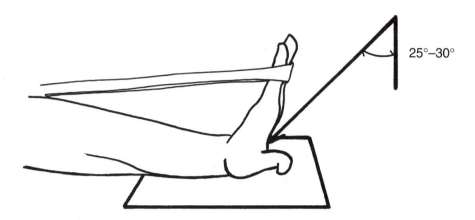

25°–30°

FIGURE 5–11. Tangential carpal canal.

NOTES
....

▶ AP FOREARM

OBJECTIVE: After practice, each student will position a patient for an AP projection of the forearm.

PATIENT PREP: Remove all jewelry from the wrist of the affected side; roll the sleeve up to midhumerus.

FILM: 11 in. × 14 in. or 10 in. × 12 in. masked lengthwise, or 7 in. × 17 in. lengthwise.

TASK ANALYSIS		CORRECTLY PERFORMED?	
MAJOR STEPS	KEY INFORMATION	YES	NO

MAJOR STEPS	KEY INFORMATION
1. Seat the patient at the end of the table with the affected side nearest the table.	The patient should be seated low enough to allow the shoulder, elbow, and wrist to lie in the same horizontal plane.
2. Position the patient's arm on the cassette with the elbow extended and the hand supinated.	The long axis of the forearm should be parallel to the long axis of the cassette.
3. Center the forearm to the unmasked half of the cassette.	Include both the wrist and elbow joints.
4. Lean the patient laterally until the forearm is in a true AP position.	Use sandbags over the hand to immobilize, if necessary.
5. Direct the central ray perpendicular to the cassette through the midpoint of the forearm.	
6. Collimate to include soft tissue and at least 1 in. of the distal humerus and proximal carpals; use gonadal shielding.	

CRITICAL ANATOMY: Shafts of the radius and ulna, radial head and neck, styloid processes of the radius and ulna, and head of the ulna.

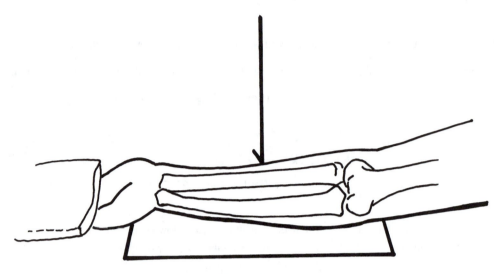

FIGURE 5–12. AP forearm.

NOTES

▶ LATERAL FOREARM

OBJECTIVE: After practice, each student will position a patient for a lateral projection of the forearm.

PATIENT PREP: Remove all jewelry from the wrist of the affected side; roll the sleeve up to midhumerus.

FILM: 11 in. × 14 in. or 10 in. × 12 in. masked lengthwise, or 7 in. × 17 in. lengthwise.

TASK ANALYSIS		CORRECTLY PERFORMED?	
MAJOR STEPS	KEY INFORMATION	YES	NO
1. Seat the patient at the end of the table with the affected side nearest the table.	The patient should be seated low enough to allow the shoulder, elbow, and wrist to lie in the same horizontal plane.		
2. Flex the elbow 90°.			
3. Position the forearm in the lateral position on the cassette.	The epicondyles of the distal humerus should be superimposed.		
4. Center the forearm to the unmasked half of the cassette.	The long axis of the forearm should be parallel to the cassette.		
5. Adjust the hand and wrist to the true lateral position.	Maintain a 90° elbow flexion with the shoulder, elbow, and wrist in the same plane.		
6. Direct the central ray perpendicular to the cassette through the midpoint of the forearm.			
7. Collimate to include soft tissue and at least 1 in. of the distal humerus and proximal carpals; use gonadal shielding.			

CRITICAL ANATOMY: Shafts of the ulna and radius, humeral epicondyles superimposed, olecranon process, trochlear notch, and radial tuberosity directed anteriorly.

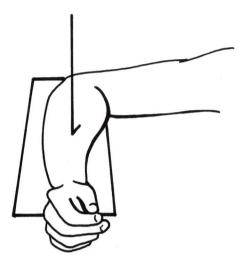

FIGURE 5–13. Lateral forearm.

NOTES
....

EVALUATOR SIGNATURE _____   DATE _____

▶ AP ELBOW

OBJECTIVE: After practice, each student will position a patient for an AP projection of the elbow.

PATIENT PREP: Roll the sleeve up to midhumerus.

FILM: 10 in. × 12 in. masked crosswise or 8 in. × 10 in. lengthwise.

TASK ANALYSIS		CORRECTLY PERFORMED?	
MAJOR STEPS	KEY INFORMATION	YES	NO
1. Seat the patient at the end of the table with the affected side nearest the table.	The patient should be seated low enough to allow the shoulder, elbow, and wrist to lie in the same horizontal plane.		
2. Position the patient's arm on the cassette with the elbow extended and the hand supinated.	The long axis of the arm must be parallel to the cassette.		
3. Center the elbow joint to the unmasked half of the cassette.			
4. Lean the patient laterally until the forearm is in true AP position.	Palpate the epicondyles of the humerus to assess positioning accuracy; use sandbags to immobilize, if necessary.		
5. Direct the central ray perpendicular to the cassette through the elbow joint.			
6. Collimate to include soft tissue and at least 2 to 3 in. of the distal humerus and proximal radius and ulna; use gonadal shielding.			

NOTE: *The olecranon process should be projected over the olecranon fossa.*

CRITICAL ANATOMY: Humeral epicondyles and condyles, trochlea, capitulum, and the radial head and neck.

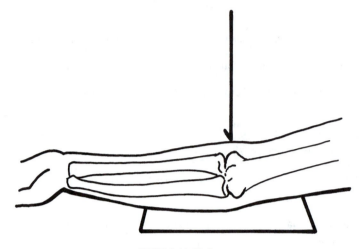

FIGURE 5–14. AP elbow.

NOTES

EVALUATOR SIGNATURE _____ DATE _____

▶ MEDIAL (INTERNAL) OBLIQUE ELBOW

OBJECTIVE: After practice, each student will position a patient for an internal oblique projection of the elbow.

PATIENT PREP: Roll the sleeve up to midhumerus.

FILM: 10 in. × 12 in. masked crosswise or 8 in. × 10 in. lengthwise.

TASK ANALYSIS		CORRECTLY PERFORMED?	
MAJOR STEPS	KEY INFORMATION	YES	NO

1. Seat the patient at the end of the table with the affected side nearest the table.	The patient should be seated low enough to allow the shoulder, elbow, and wrist to lie in the same horizontal plane.		
2. Position the patient's arm on the cassette with the elbow extended and the hand supinated.	The long axis of the arm should be parallel to the cassette.		
3. Center the elbow joint to the unmasked half of the cassette.			
4. Internally rotate the entire arm so a line passing through the humeral epicondyles is at a 40–45° angle with the film plane.	The hand may be pronated for support; a sandbag may be used for immobilization.		
5. Direct the central ray perpendicular to the cassette through the elbow joint.			
6. Collimate to include soft tissue and at least 2 to 3 in. of the distal humerus and proximal radius and ulna; use gonadal shielding.			

CRITICAL ANATOMY: Coronoid process.

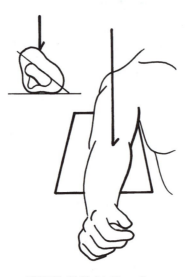

FIGURE 5–15. Medial oblique elbow.

NOTES

▶ LATERAL (EXTERNAL) OBLIQUE ELBOW

OBJECTIVE: After practice, each student will position a patient for an external oblique projection of the elbow.

PATIENT PREP: Roll the sleeve up to midhumerus.

FILM: 10 in. × 12 in. masked crosswise or 8 in. × 10 in. lengthwise.

TASK ANALYSIS		CORRECTLY PERFORMED?	
MAJOR STEPS	KEY INFORMATION	YES	NO

1. Seat the patient at the end of the table with the affected side nearest the table.	The patient should be seated low enough to allow the shoulder, elbow, and wrist to lie in the same horizontal plane.		
2. Position the patient's arm on the cassette with the elbow extended and the hand supinated.	The long axis of the arm should be parallel to the cassette.		
3. Center the elbow joint to the unmasked half of the cassette.			
4. Externally rotate the entire arm so a line passing through the humeral epicondyles is at a 40° angle with the film plane.	Lean the patient backward and gently depress the shoulder until the position is achieved; the position will be uncomfortable. Use sponges and sandbags to support and immobilize, if necessary.		
5. Direct the central ray perpendicular to the cassette through the elbow joint.			
6. Collimate to include soft tissue and at least 2 to 3 in. of the distal humerus and proximal radius and ulna; use gonadal shielding.			

CRITICAL ANATOMY: Proximal radioulnar joint, radial head, radial notch of the ulna, and radial tuberosity free of superimposition.

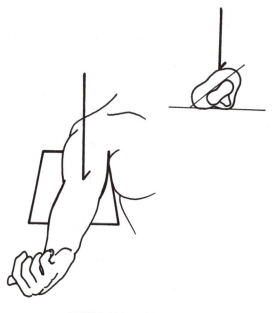

FIGURE 5–16. Lateral oblique elbow.

NOTES
....

▶ LATERAL ELBOW

OBJECTIVE: After practice, each student will position a patient for a lateral projection of the elbow.

PATIENT PREP: Roll the sleeve up to midhumerus.

FILM: 10 in. × 12 in. masked crosswise or 8 in. × 10 in. lengthwise.

TASK ANALYSIS		CORRECTLY PERFORMED?	
MAJOR STEPS	KEY INFORMATION	YES	NO
1. Seat the patient at the end of the table with the affected side nearest the table.	The patient should be seated low enough to allow the shoulder, elbow, and wrist to lie in the same horizontal plane.		
2. Flex the elbow 90°.			
3. Position the forearm in the lateral position with the elbow on the cassette.	The epicondyles of the distal humerus should be superimposed.		
4. Center the elbow joint to the unmasked half of the cassette.	The long axis of the humerus should be parallel to the long axis of the cassette field.		
5. Adjust the hand and wrist to the true lateral position.	Maintain a 90° elbow flexion with the shoulder, elbow, and wrist in the same plane; use sandbags to immobilize, if necessary.		
6. Direct the central ray perpendicular to the cassette through the elbow joint.			
7. Collimate to include soft tissue and at least 2 to 3 in. of the distal humerus and proximal radius and ulna; use gonadal shielding.			

CRITICAL ANATOMY: Olecranon process, trochlear notch, and radial tuberosity directed anteriorly.

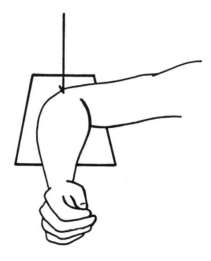

FIGURE 5–17. Lateral elbow.

NOTES

▶ AXIAL LATERAL ELBOW

OBJECTIVE: After practice, each student will position a patient for an axial projection of the elbow in the lateral
                  position.

PATIENT PREP: Roll the sleeve up to midhumerus.

FILM: 8 in. × 10 in. lengthwise or 9 in. × 9 in.

TASK ANALYSIS		CORRECTLY PERFORMED?	
MAJOR STEPS	KEY INFORMATION	YES	NO

1. Seat the patient at the end of the table with the affected side nearest the table.	The patient should be seated low enough to allow the shoulder, elbow, and wrist to lie in the same horizontal plane.		
2. Flex the elbow 90°.			
3. Position the forearm and elbow in the lateral position.	The humeral epicondyles should be perpendicular to the cassette.		
4. Center the elbow joint to the cassette.			
5. Adjust the hand and wrist to the true lateral position.	Maintain a 90° elbow flexion with the shoulder, elbow, and wrist in the same plane; use a sandbag to immobilize.		
6. Direct the central ray at a 45° angle to the humerus through the elbow joint.			
7. Adjust the centering of the cassette to coincide with the central ray.			
8. Collimate to include soft tissue and at least 2 in. of the distal humerus and proximal radius and ulna; use gonadal shielding.			

NOTE: *This projection may be requested in cases of trauma to demonstrate a fracture of the radial head.*

CRITICAL ANATOMY: Elongated view of the radial head, free of superimposition.

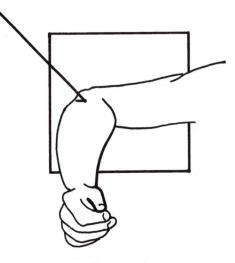

FIGURE 5–18. Axial lateral elbow.

NOTES
....

▶ AP HUMERUS

OBJECTIVE: After practice, each student will position a patient for an AP projection of the humerus.

PATIENT PREP: Remove all clothing and jewelry from the waist up; gown patient.

FILM: 14 in. × 17 in. or 7 in. × 17 in. lengthwise, grid or non-grid.

TASK ANALYSIS		CORRECTLY PERFORMED?	
MAJOR STEPS	KEY INFORMATION	YES	NO
1. Position the patient supine on the table.	The body should be aligned to the long axis of the table without rotation. *Note:* Because shoulder and arm injuries may be extremely painful, the erect position may be preferred and performed more quickly and easily.		
2. Center the affected arm to the table.			
3. Elevate the unaffected side with a small sandbag or sponge to place the affected arm in contact with the table.			
4. Supinate the hand.	The epicondyles should be parallel to the film plane. Use sandbags to immobilize.		
5. Position the cassette to include the shoulder and elbow joints.	The long axis of the humerus should be parallel to the long axis of the cassette. Large-breasted women may have to hold the breast out of the way with the opposite hand.		
6. Direct the central ray perpendicular to the midhumerus.			
7. Collimate to include soft tissue and elbow and shoulder joints; use gonadal shielding.			

CRITICAL ANATOMY: Greater tubercle, humeral head, medial and lateral epicondyles and condyles, and anatomical and surgical necks.

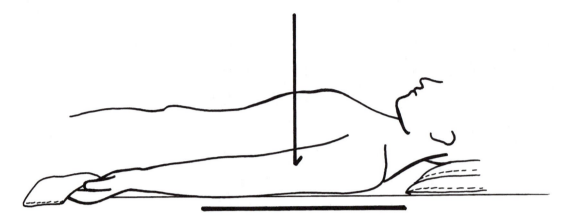

FIGURE 5–19. AP humerus.

NOTES
....

► LATERAL HUMERUS

OBJECTIVE: After practice, each student will position a patient for a lateral projection of the humerus.

PATIENT PREP: Remove all clothing and jewelry from the waist up; gown patient.

FILM: 14 in. × 17 in. or 7 in. × 17 in. lengthwise, grid or non-grid.

TASK ANALYSIS		CORRECTLY PERFORMED?	
MAJOR STEPS	KEY INFORMATION	YES	NO
1. Position the patient supine on the table.	The body should be aligned to the long axis of the table without rotation. *Note:* Because shoulder and arm injuries may be extremely painful, the erect position may be preferred and performed more quickly and easily.		
2. Center the affected arm to the table.			
3. Elevate the unaffected side with a small sandbag or sponge to place the affected arm in contact with the table.			
4. Abduct the arm slightly and internally rotate the entire arm so the back of the hand rests against the side of the hip.	The humeral epicondyles should be perpendicular to the film plane. Use a sandbag to immobilize.		
5. Position the cassette to include the shoulder and elbow joints.	The long axis of the humerus should be parallel to the long axis of the cassette when possible. Large-breasted women may have to hold the breast out of the way with the opposite hand.		
6. Direct the central ray perpendicular to the midhumerus.			
7. Collimate to include soft tissue and elbow and shoulder joints; use gonadal shielding.			

CRITICAL ANATOMY: Lesser tubercle.

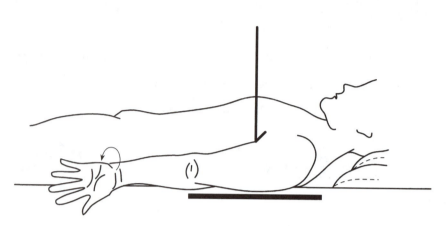

FIGURE 5–20. Lateral humerus.

NOTES

EVALUATOR SIGNATURE _____ DATE _____

▶ TRANSTHORACIC LATERAL HUMERUS: NEUTRAL POSITION (TRAUMA)

OBJECTIVE: After practice, each student will position a patient for a transthoracic lateral projection of the humerus with the arm in the neutral position.

PATIENT PREP: Remove all clothing and jewelry from the waist up; gown patient.

FILM: 10 in. × 12 in. lengthwise, grid.

TASK ANALYSIS		CORRECTLY PERFORMED?	
MAJOR STEPS	KEY INFORMATION	YES	NO
1. Assist the patient into the erect lateral position in front of the vertical grid device with the affected side nearest the film.			
2. Instruct the patient to raise the unaffected arm and rest the forearm on the head.	The unaffected shoulder should be elevated as much as possible to separate the shoulders and prevent superimposition.		
3. Center the cassette to the surgical neck of the affected side.	The top of the cassette should be 1 1/2 to 2 in. above the top of the shoulder.		
4. Adjust the rotation of the body to project the humerus between the spine and the sternum.			
5. Direct the central ray perpendicular to the midpoint of the cassette.			
6. Collimate to include the humerus and glenohumeral joint; use gonadal shielding.			
7. Make the exposure during either: a. Suspended full *inspiration,* or b. Slow, deep breathing.	A long exposure time is needed to blur lung detail.		

CRITICAL ANATOMY: Head and neck of the humerus, acromion process, and coracoid process.

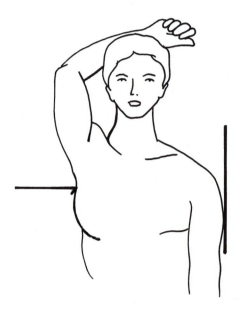

FIGURE 5–21. Transthoracic lateral humerus.

NOTES

EVALUATOR SIGNATURE _____ DATE _____

SHOULDER GIRDLE

▶ AP SHOULDER IN EXTERNAL ROTATION

OBJECTIVE: After practice, each student will position a patient for an AP projection of the shoulder in external rotation.

PATIENT PREP: Remove all clothing and jewelry from the waist up; gown patient.

FILM: 10 in. × 12 in. crosswise or lengthwise (depending on department routine), grid.

TASK ANALYSIS		CORRECTLY PERFORMED?	
MAJOR STEPS	KEY INFORMATION	YES	NO
1. Position the patient supine on the table.	The body should be aligned to the long axis of the table without rotation. If a fracture is suspected, the examination should be performed with the patient upright against a vertical grid device.		
2. Center the coracoid process of the affected shoulder to the midline of the grid device.			
3. Slightly rotate the patient toward the affected side to place the shoulder parallel with the film plane.	Rotation will overcome the curve in the back and obliquity of the shoulder structures. Use a sponge or sandbag to support the unaffected side.		
4. Supinate the hand.	The epicondyles should be parallel to the film plane. Use a sandbag across the forearm or hand to immobilize, if necessary.		
5. Direct the central ray perpendicular to the coracoid process.			
6. Center the cassette to the central ray.			
7. Turn the patient's head away from the side being examined.	Rotating the head places the eyes further away from the central ray.		
8. Collimate to include the clavicle and proximal third of the humerus; use gonadal shielding.	Lead masking may be positioned on the table above the shoulder to reduce the amount of scatter reaching the film and improve image quality. When doing this, the lead marker should be in the lower lateral corner of the cassette.		
9. Make the exposure during suspended respiration.			

CRITICAL ANATOMY: Greater tubercle of the humerus in profile; the relationship of the glenohumeral joint and the shoulder and humerus in anatomical position.

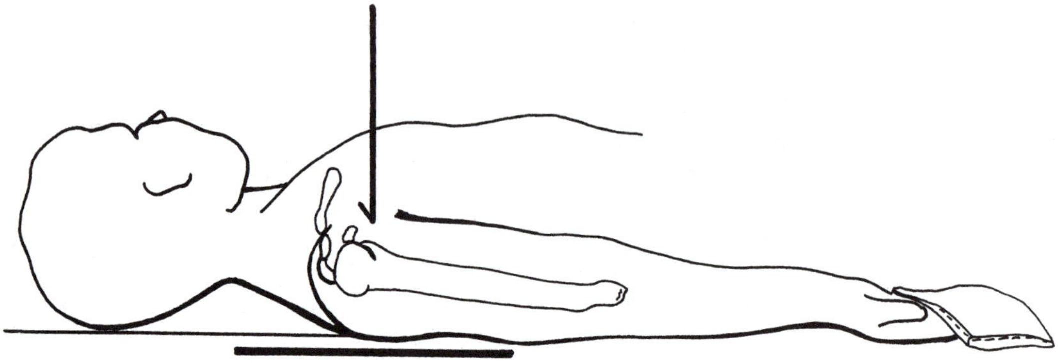

FIGURE 6–1. AP shoulder, external rotation.

NOTES

EVALUATOR SIGNATURE ______________________ DATE ____________

► AP SHOULDER IN INTERNAL ROTATION

OBJECTIVE: After practice, each student will position a patient for an AP projection of the shoulder in internal rotation.

PATIENT PREP: Remove all clothing and jewelry from the waist up; gown patient.

FILM: 10 in. × 12 in. crosswise or lengthwise (depending on department routine), grid.

TASK ANALYSIS		CORRECTLY PERFORMED?	
MAJOR STEPS	KEY INFORMATION	YES	NO
1. Position the patient supine on the table.	The body should be aligned to the long axis of the table without rotation. If a fracture is suspected, the examination should be performed with the patient upright against a vertical grid device.		
2. Center the coracoid process of the affected shoulder to the midline of the grid device.			
3. Slightly rotate the patient toward the affected side to place the shoulder parallel with the film plane.	Rotation will overcome the curve in the back and obliquity of the shoulder structures. Use a sponge or sandbag to support the unaffected side.		
4. Rotate the arm internally, flexing the elbow slightly and placing the back of the hand against the hip.	The humerus will be in the lateral position with the epicondyles perpendicular with the film plane. Use a sandbag against the forearm or hand for immobilization, if necessary.		
5. Direct the central ray perpendicular to the coracoid process.			
6. Center the cassette to the central ray.			
7. Turn the patient's head away from the side being examined.	Rotating the head places the eyes further away from the central ray.		
8. Collimate to include the clavicle and proximal third of the humerus; use gonadal shielding.	Lead masking may be positioned on the table above the shoulder to reduce the amount of scatter reaching the film and improve image quality. When doing this, the lead marker should be in the lower lateral corner of the cassette.		
9. Make the exposure during suspended respiration.			

CRITICAL ANATOMY: Lesser tubercle in profile near glenoid fossa; glenohumeral joint relationship.

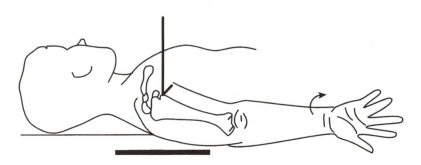

FIGURE 6–2. AP shoulder, internal rotation.

NOTES
....

► INFEROSUPERIOR AXIAL SHOULDER JOINT (LAWRENCE POSITION)

OBJECTIVE: After practice, each student will position a patient for an inferosuperior axial projection (axillary view) of the shoulder in the Lawrence position.

PATIENT PREP: Remove all clothing and jewelry from the waist up; gown patient.

FILM: 10 in. × 12 in. or 8 in. × 10 in. crosswise, grid or non-grid; support vertically.

TASK ANALYSIS		CORRECTLY PERFORMED?	
MAJOR STEPS	KEY INFORMATION	YES	NO

1. Position the patient supine on the table.

2. Elevate the head, affected shoulder, and upper thorax 3 to 4 in. using sponges or other suitable support.

3. Abduct the patient's arm 90° to the long axis of the body (or as far as the patient will permit). — This may be very painful; move the patient slowly; *do not force movement.*

4. While keeping the arm in external rotation, adjust the forearm and hand to a comfortable position. — Use sandbags to support the arm.

5. Turn the patient's head away from the side being examined. — Rotation of the head removes the eyes from the primary beam and allows for better placement of the cassette.

6. Place the cassette vertically above the shoulder and as close as possible to the neck. — Use sandbags or a cassette holder to support the cassette.

7. Direct the central ray horizontally through the axilla to the acromioclavicular joint. — The degree of medial angulation depends on the degree of abduction of the arm; 30–35° with lateral body surface for 90° abduction and 20° for ≤60° abduction. The cassette should be adjusted so it is perpendicular to the central ray.

8. Collimate to include the glenoid cavity, acromion, coracoid process, and surgical neck; use gonadal shielding.

9. Make the exposure during suspended respiration.

CRITICAL ANATOMY: Glenohumeral joint.

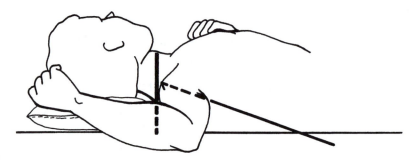

FIGURE 6–3. Inferosuperior axial shoulder joint.

NOTES
....

▶ PA OBLIQUE "Y" SHOULDER JOINT

OBJECTIVE: After practice, each student will position a patient for a "Y" view of the shoulder joint.

PATIENT PREP: Remove all clothing and jewelry from the waist up; gown patient.

FILM: 10 in. × 12 in. lengthwise, grid.

TASK ANALYSIS		CORRECTLY PERFORMED?	
MAJOR STEPS	KEY INFORMATION	YES	NO
1. Assist the patient to the anterior oblique position in front of the upright grid device with the affected side nearest the upright device.	The projection may be obtained with the patient recumbent if the patient is unable to sit on a stool or stand.		
2. Center the humeral head of the affected side to the midline of the grid device.			
3. Adjust the rotation of the body so the midcoronal plane forms a 45–60° angle with the film plane.	The plane of the affected scapula should be perpendicular to the film plane.		
4. Position the affected arm comfortably at the patient's side.			
5. Direct the central ray horizontally through the vertebral border of the scapula to the glenohumeral joint.	The upper border of the cassette should be approximately 1 1/2 in. above the top of the shoulder.		
6. Center the cassette to the central ray.			
7. Collimate to include the acromion, coracoid process, and surgical neck of humerus; use gonadal shielding.			
8. Make the exposure during suspended respiration.			

CRITICAL ANATOMY: Glenohumeral joint, acromion, and coracoid process.

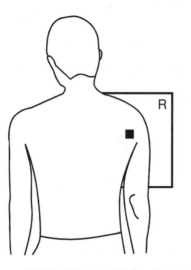

FIGURE 6–4. PA oblique "Y" view of the shoulder.

NOTES
....

EVALUATOR SIGNATURE _____ DATE _____

► AP CLAVICLE

OBJECTIVE: After practice, each student will position a patient for an AP projection of the clavicle.

PATIENT PREP: Remove all clothing and jewelry from the waist up; gown patient.

FILM: 10 in. × 12 in. crosswise, grid.

MAJOR STEPS	KEY INFORMATION	YES	NO
1. Position the patient supine on the table.	The body should be aligned to the long axis of the table without rotation.		
2. Center the midclavicle to the midline of the grid device.			
3. Position the patient's arms at the sides and adjust the shoulders to lie in the same transverse plane.			
4. Direct the central ray perpendicular to the midpoint of the clavicle.	If the patient's head is on a pillow, make sure the edge of the pillow will not be under the anatomy.		
5. Center the cassette to the central ray.	The cassette should be centered to the level of the coracoid process.		
6. Turn the head away from the side being examined.	Rotating the head places the eyes further away from the central ray.		
7. Collimate to include the clavicle and associated joints; use gonadal shielding.			
8. Make the exposure during suspended *inspiration*.			

TASK ANALYSIS / CORRECTLY PERFORMED?

NOTE: *Although the PA projection is preferred to reduce magnification, the AP projection is generally used to prevent additional injury.*

CRITICAL ANATOMY: Body and sternal and acromial extremities of the clavicle.

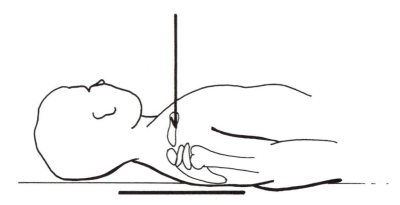

FIGURE 6–5. AP clavicle.

NOTES
....

▶ AP AXIAL CLAVICLE

OBJECTIVE: After practice, each student will position a patient for an AP axial projection of the clavicle.

PATIENT PREP: Remove all clothing and jewelry from the waist up; gown patient.

FILM: 10 in. × 12 in. crosswise, grid.

TASK ANALYSIS		CORRECTLY PERFORMED?	
MAJOR STEPS	KEY INFORMATION	YES	NO
1. Position the patient supine on the table.	The body should be aligned to the long axis of the table without rotation.		
2. Center the midclavicle to the midline of the grid device.			
3. Position the patient's arms at the sides and adjust the shoulders to lie in the same transverse plane.			
4. Direct the central ray 25–30° cephalad to the midclavicle.	The degree of angulation may be as little as 15° or as much as 45°, depending on department routine and thickness of the chest. A thin chest will require more angulation to project the clavicle above the thorax.		
5. Center the cassette to the central ray.	If the patient's head is on a pillow, make sure the edge of the pillow will not be under the anatomy.		
6. Turn the head away from the side being examined.	Rotating the head places the eyes further away from the central ray.		
7. Collimate to include the clavicle and associated joints; use gonadal shielding.			
8. Make the exposure during suspended *inspiration*.			

CRITICAL ANATOMY: Body and sternal and acromial extremities of the clavicle.

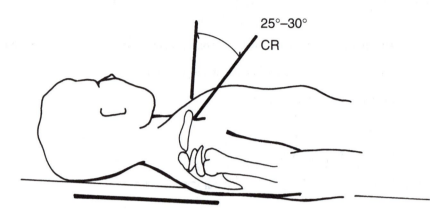

FIGURE 6–6. AP axial clavicle.

NOTES

▶ AP SCAPULA

OBJECTIVE: After practice, each student will position a patient for an AP projection of the scapula.

PATIENT PREP: Remove all clothing and jewelry from the waist up; gown patient.

FILM: 10 in. × 12 in. lengthwise, grid.

TASK ANALYSIS		CORRECTLY PERFORMED?	
MAJOR STEPS	KEY INFORMATION	YES	NO
1. Position the patient supine on the table.	The body should be aligned to the long axis of the table, without rotation.		
2. Center the coracoid process to the midline of the table.	A point halfway between the midline of the body and the lateral border of the shoulder should be centered to the table.		
3. Abduct the arm 90° to the long axis of the body.	Abducting the arm will move the scapula laterally.		
4. Flex the elbow and supinate the hand.	The hand may be supported with sandbags near the patient's head.		
5. Direct the central ray perpendicular to the midscapula.			
6. Center the cassette to the central ray.	The upper border of the cassette should be approximately 1 1/2 in. above the shoulder.		
7. Collimate to include the scapula and shoulder joint; use gonadal shielding.			
8. Make the exposure during *quiet breathing*.	Quiet breathing will blur the lung detail.		

CRITICAL ANATOMY: Acromion process, coracoid process, scapular notch, glenoid fossa, inferior and superior angles, and axillary and vertebral borders.

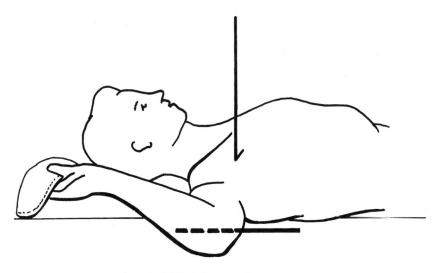

FIGURE 6–7. AP scapula.

NOTES

▶ LATERAL SCAPULA

OBJECTIVE: After practice, each student will position a patient for a lateral projection of the scapula.

PATIENT PREP: Remove all clothing and jewelry from the waist up; gown patient.

FILM: 10 in. × 12 in. lengthwise, grid.

TASK ANALYSIS		CORRECTLY PERFORMED?	
MAJOR STEPS	KEY INFORMATION	YES	NO

1. Assist the patient to the anterior oblique position in front of the upright grid device with the affected side nearest the upright device.	The projection may be obtained with the patient recumbent if the patient is unable to sit on a stool or stand.		
2. Center the affected scapula to the midline of the grid device.			
3. Position the arm according to the area of the scapula to be demonstrated: a. *Body:* Flex the elbow and rest the back of the hand on the back of the waist or front of the chest. b. *Acromion and coracoid processes:* Extend the arm upward and place the forearm on the head. c. *Glenohumeral joint:* Position the arm beside the body so the humerus and the wing of the scapula are superimposed.			
4. Palpate the axillary and vertebral borders between the thumb and fingers and adjust the body rotation to place the wing of the scapula perpendicular to the plane of the cassette.	Palpation is difficult when patients are obese or muscular.		
5. Center the cassette so the upper border is approximately 1 1/2 in. above the top of the shoulder.			
6. Direct the central ray perpendicular to the center of the cassette through the vertebral border of the scapula.			
7. Collimate to include the scapula and shoulder joint; use gonadal shielding.			

Continued

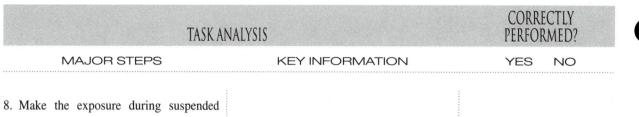

TASK ANALYSIS		CORRECTLY PERFORMED?	
MAJOR STEPS	KEY INFORMATION	YES	NO

8. Make the exposure during suspended respiration.

CRITICAL ANATOMY: Acromion process, coracoid process, scapular spine, inferior angle, costal and dorsal surfaces, and the body of the scapula.

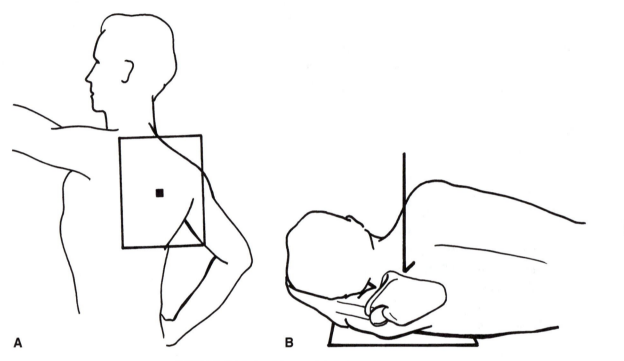

A   B

FIGURE 6–8. **A.** Lateral scapula, erect. **B.** Lateral scapula, recumbent.

NOTES

EVALUATOR SIGNATURE _____ DATE _____

► AP ACROMIOCLAVICULAR JOINTS: WITH & WITHOUT WEIGHTS

OBJECTIVE: After practice, each student will position a patient for bilateral frontal projections of the acromio-clavicular articulations with and without weights.

PATIENT PREP: Remove all clothing and jewelry from the waist up; gown patient.

FILM: 7 in. × 17 in. crosswise or 2–8 in. × 10 in. crosswise if necessary for large patients, grid or non-grid.

TASK ANALYSIS		CORRECTLY PERFORMED?	
MAJOR STEPS	KEY INFORMATION	YES	NO
1. Assist the patient to the seated or standing AP position in front of an upright cassette holder.	Because dislocation of the acromioclavicular joint tends to reduce itself in the recumbent position, this projection must be performed upright.		
2. Center the cassette to the level of the acromioclavicular joints.	If the patient is too broad for one crosswise cassette, use one small cassette for each joint (four exposures instead of two).		
3. Center the midline of the patient to the center of the cassette.	If using separate cassettes, center the acromioclavicular joint to the cassette.		
4. Instruct the patient to distribute the body weight equally on both feet.			
5. Adjust the shoulders to lie in the same transverse plane with the arms hanging unsupported at the sides.			
6. Using 72-in. SID, direct the central ray perpendicular to the midline of the body at the level of the acromioclavicular joints.	Center to the acromioclavicular joint if using small cassettes. A 72-in. SID minimizes magnification and, on most patients, permits visualization of both acromioclavicular joints on one film.		
7. Center the cassette to the central ray.			
8. Collimate to include the acromioclavicular joints; use gonadal shielding.			

Continued

TASK ANALYSIS		CORRECTLY PERFORMED?	
MAJOR STEPS	KEY INFORMATION	YES	NO

9. Take two successive exposures without changing the patient's position:
   a. One with arms hanging freely at the sides.
   b. One with equal weights suspended from each wrist.

Four exposures will be made if using small cassettes.

Instruct the patient to allow the weights to pull the shoulders downward. Sandbags may be placed in pillow cases and suspended from the wrists. *Note:* A fracture of the clavicle, shoulder, or arm *must* be ruled out before giving weights to any patient.

10. Make the exposure during suspended *expiration*.

CRITICAL ANATOMY: Acromioclavicular joints.

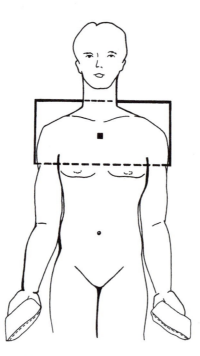

FIGURE 6–9. Bilateral AP acromioclavicular joints, with weights.

EVALUATOR SIGNATURE _____ DATE _____

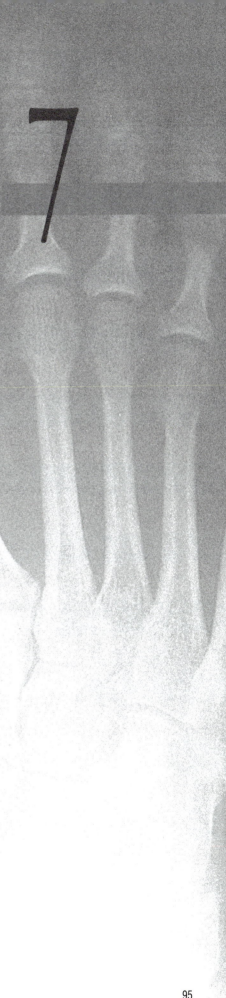

LOWER LIMB (EXTREMITY)

▶ PA PATELLA

▶ TANGENTIAL PATELLA & PATELLOFEMORAL JOINT ("SUNRISE," "SKYLINE," SETTEGAST METHOD)

▶ AP FEMUR

▶ LATERAL FEMUR

► AP & MEDIAL OBLIQUE TOES

OBJECTIVE: After practice, each student will position a patient for AP and medial oblique projections of the toes.

PATIENT PREP: Remove the shoe and sock from the affected foot.

FILM: 8 in. × 10 in. or 9 in. × 9 in. masked crosswise.

TASK ANALYSIS		CORRECTLY PERFORMED?	
MAJOR STEPS	KEY INFORMATION	YES	NO

MAJOR STEPS	KEY INFORMATION		
1. Position the patient supine or seated on the table.			

2. Flex the knee of the affected side until the sole of the foot rests firmly on the unmasked half of the cassette.
  a. *AP:* Rest the foot on the plantar surface of the foot.
  b. *Medial oblique:* Rest the foot on the plantar surface and rotate the leg internally until the sole of the foot forms a 30° angle with the film plane.
	The foot should be in a true AP position.		

3. Center the 2nd metatarsophalangeal joint to the unmasked half of the cassette.			
4. Direct the central ray perpendicular to the cassette through the 2nd metatarsophalangeal joint.	Depending on department routine, the central ray may be directed to the individual toe of interest.		
5. Collimate to soft tissue and one half of the distal metatarsals; use gonadal shielding.			

CRITICAL ANATOMY: Phalanges, interphalangeal joints, and metatarsophalangeal joints.

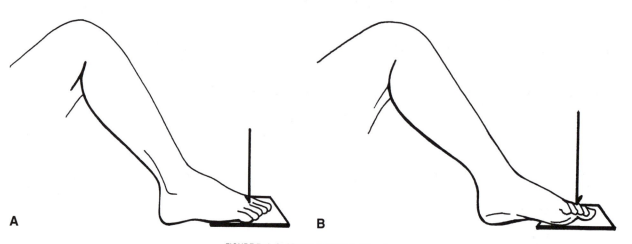

FIGURE 7–1. **A.** AP toes. **B.** Medial oblique toes.

NOTES

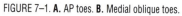

▶ TANGENTIAL METATARSOPHALANGEAL SESAMOID BONES (LEWIS METHOD)

OBJECTIVE: After practice, each student will position a patient for a tangential projection of the metatarsophalangeal sesamoid bones using the Lewis method.

PATIENT PREP: Remove the shoe and sock from the affected foot.

FILM: 8 in. × 10 in., 9 in. × 9 in. or occlusal.

TASK ANALYSIS		CORRECTLY PERFORMED?	
MAJOR STEPS	KEY INFORMATION	YES	NO
1. Assist the patient to the prone position on the table.			
2. Elevate the ankle of the affected side using sandbags or other support.	Place a folded towel or small sponge under the patient's knee for comfort.		
3. Dorsiflex the foot and place the great toe on the cassette.	The ball of the foot will be perpendicular to the film plane.		
4. Center the 1st metatarsal to the midpoint of the cassette.			
5. Direct the central ray perpendicular to the 1st metatarsophalangeal joint.			
6. Collimate to soft tissue and the heads of the 1st, 2nd, and 3rd metatarsals; use gonadal shielding.			

NOTE: *This projection may also be obtained with the patient sitting and holding the toes in dorsiflexion using a strip of gauze bandage or tape.*

CRITICAL ANATOMY: Sesamoid bones.

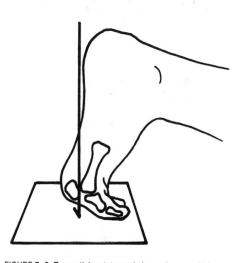

FIGURE 7–2. Tangential metatarsophalangeal sesamoid bones.

NOTES
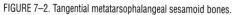

► AP (DORSOPLANTAR) FOOT

OBJECTIVE: After practice, each student will position a patient for a dorsoplantar projection of the foot.

PATIENT PREP: Remove the shoe and sock from the affected foot.

FILM: 10 in. × 12 in., masked lengthwise.

TASK ANALYSIS		CORRECTLY PERFORMED?	
MAJOR STEPS	KEY INFORMATION	YES	NO
1. Position the patient supine or seated on the table.			
2. Flex the knee of the affected side until the sole of the foot rests firmly on the table.	The patient may brace this position by flexing the opposite knee and leaning it against the knee of the affected side.		
3. Center the foot to the unmasked half of the cassette.	Position the cassette so the patient ID blocker is toward the patient and make sure the toes are included on the cassette. Use a sandbag or tape to prevent the cassette from sliding.		
4. Direct the central ray 10° cephalad to the base of the 3rd metatarsal.	The angle can vary from 5–15° depending on the arch of the foot. The angulation demonstrates the tarsal and metatarsal joint spaces.		
5. Collimate to include soft tissue, toes, and all tarsals; use gonadal shielding.			

CRITICAL ANATOMY: Phalanges, metatarsals, metatarsophalangeal joints, tarsometatarsal joints, medial and intermediate cuneiforms, and navicular.

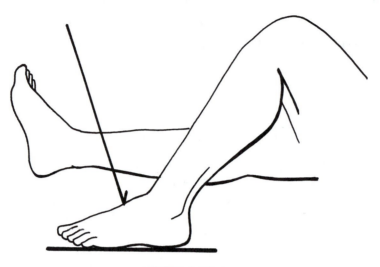

FIGURE 7–3. AP foot.

NOTES
....

▶ MEDIAL OBLIQUE FOOT

OBJECTIVE: After practice, each student will position a patient for a medial oblique projection of the foot.

PATIENT PREP: Remove the shoe and sock from the affected foot.

FILM: 10 in. × 12 in. masked lengthwise.

TASK ANALYSIS		CORRECTLY PERFORMED?	
MAJOR STEPS	KEY INFORMATION	YES	NO

MAJOR STEPS	KEY INFORMATION
1. Position the patient supine or seated on the table.	
2. Flex the knee of the affected side until the sole of the foot rests firmly on the table.	
3. Rotate the leg internally until the sole of the foot forms an angle of 30° with the cassette.	The patient may brace this position by using the opposite leg. As much as a 45° angle may be necessary for feet with high arches.
4. Adjust the foot so the base of the 3rd metatarsal is centered to the unmasked half of the cassette.	Use a sandbag or tape to keep the cassette from sliding on the table top.
5. Direct the central ray perpendicular to the cassette through the base of the 3rd metatarsal.	
6. Collimate to include soft tissue, toes, and all tarsals; use gonadal shielding.	

CRITICAL ANATOMY: Cuboid and lateral cuneiform free of superimposition, navicular, talus, calcaneus, metatarsals, sinus tarsi, and the phalanges.

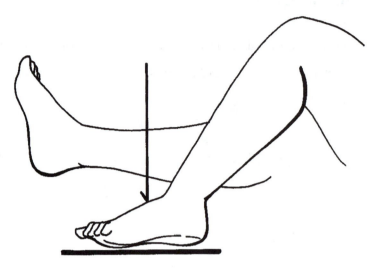

FIGURE 7–4. Medial oblique foot.

NOTES
....

EVALUATOR SIGNATURE _____ DATE _____

► LATERAL FOOT

OBJECTIVE: After practice, each student will position a patient for a lateral projection of the foot.

PATIENT PREP: Remove the shoe and sock from the affected foot.

FILM: 10 in. × 12 in. lengthwise or angled.

TASK ANALYSIS		CORRECTLY PERFORMED?	
MAJOR STEPS	KEY INFORMATION	YES	NO
1. Position the patient in the lateral recumbent position with the lateral surface of the affected foot down.	The lateral projection may also be obtained with the medial surface nearest the film.		
2. Adjust the leg so the plantar surface of the foot is perpendicular to the plane of the cassette.	Elevating the knee on a sandbag or other support so that the patella is perpendicular to the cassette will help place the foot in the correct position. Neither the calcaneus nor the metatarsals should be elevated from the cassette.		
3. Center the cassette to the midfoot.	The central ray will enter approximately at the tarsometatarsal joints.		
4. Direct the central ray perpendicular to the center of the cassette.			
5. Collimate to include all soft tissue and 1 in. of the distal tibia and fibula; use gonadal shielding.	Rotate the tube or collimator to coincide with the long axis of the foot to allow for maximum collimation.		

CRITICAL ANATOMY: Calcaneus, talus, and navicular.

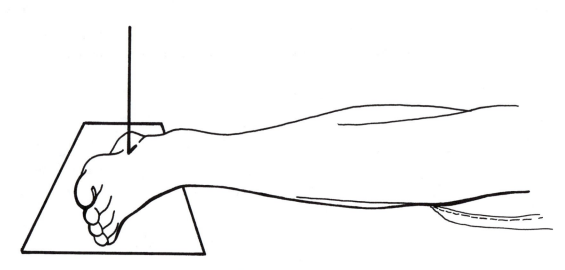

FIGURE 7–5. Lateral foot.

NOTES

▶ AXIAL PLANTODORSAL CALCANEUS (OS CALCIS)

OBJECTIVE: After practice, each student will position a patient for a plantodorsal projection of the calcaneus (os calcis).

PATIENT PREP: Remove the shoe and sock from the affected foot.

FILM: 8 in. × 10 in. lengthwise, or 8 in. × 10 in. or 10 in. × 12 in. masked crosswise.

TASK ANALYSIS		CORRECTLY PERFORMED?	
MAJOR STEPS	KEY INFORMATION	YES	NO
1. Seat the patient on the table with the legs parallel to the long axis of the table.			
2. Center the cassette to the malleoli of the ankle.			
3. Position a long strip of cloth around the ball of the foot and have the patient pull back on it in order to hold the foot in 90° dorsiflexion.	If the patient cannot flex the ankle enough to place the plantar surface of the foot perpendicular to the table, sponges can be used to raise the leg for accurate positioning.		
4. Direct the central ray 40° cephalad to the midplantar surface at the level of the base of the 5th metatarsal.	If the dorsiflexion is beyond 90°, a smaller angle should be used; if the foot is plantar flexed, a greater angle is required.		
5. Collimate to include soft tissue of the calcaneus and proximal metatarsals; use gonadal shielding.			

NOTE: *This projection may also be obtained with the patient prone and the central ray directed caudally.*

CRITICAL ANATOMY: Calcaneus and subtalar joint.

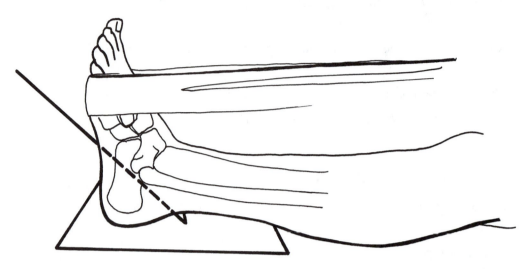

FIGURE 7–6. Axial plantodorsal calcaneus.

NOTES
....

▶ LATERAL CALCANEUS (OS CALCIS)

OBJECTIVE: After practice, each student will position a patient for a lateral projection of the calcaneus (os cal-
               cis).

PATIENT PREP: Remove the shoe and sock from the affected foot.

FILM: 8 in. × 10 in. or 10 in. × 12 in. masked crosswise.

TASK ANALYSIS		CORRECTLY PERFORMED?	
MAJOR STEPS	KEY INFORMATION	YES	NO
1. Assist the patient to the lateral recumbent position on the table with the lateral surface of the affected heel down.	The lower leg should be parallel with the film plane. This projection may also be obtained with the medial surface nearest the film.		
2. Adjust the cassette so the long axis is parallel to the plantar surface of the heel.			
3. With the foot dorsiflexed 90°, position the foot so the plantar surface is perpendicular to the film plane.	Neither the calcaneus nor the metatarsals should be elevated from the cassette.		
4. Center the midpoint of the calcaneus, about 1 to 1 1/2 in. distal to the medial malleolus, to the cassette.			
5. Direct the central ray perpendicular to the cassette through the heel.			
6. Collimate to include soft tissue of the calcaneus and the ankle joint; use gonadal shielding.			

CRITICAL ANATOMY: Calcaneus and subtalar joint.

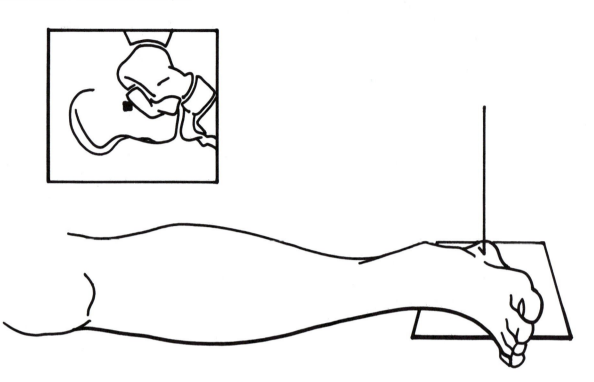

FIGURE 7–7. Lateral calcaneus.

NOTES

► AP ANKLE

OBJECTIVE: After practice, each student will position a patient for an AP projection of the ankle.

PATIENT PREP: Remove the shoe and sock from the affected foot; roll the pant leg up.

FILM: 10 in. × 12 in. masked crosswise.

TASK ANALYSIS		CORRECTLY PERFORMED?	
MAJOR STEPS	KEY INFORMATION	YES	NO
1. Seat the patient on the table with the legs parallel to the long axis of the table.	The knee of the unaffected side can be flexed to relieve strain and make the patient more comfortable.		
2. Center the ankle joint to the unmasked half of the cassette.	The cassette may be positioned off-centered lengthwise to both the ankle joint and the central ray to include more of the distal lower leg.		
3. Dorsiflex the ankle so the foot and leg are at a 90° angle.	The toes should point straight up. This position may be painful; move the patient slowly and immobilize with sandbags, if necessary.		
4. Direct the central ray perpendicular to the ankle joint at a point midway between the malleoli.	The ankle joint is about 1/2 in. above the bottom of the malleoli.		
5. Collimate to include the proximal talus, medial and lateral malleoli, and distal fourth of the lower leg; use gonadal shielding.			

CRITICAL ANATOMY: Medial and lateral malleoli, proximal talus, and tibiotalar joint.

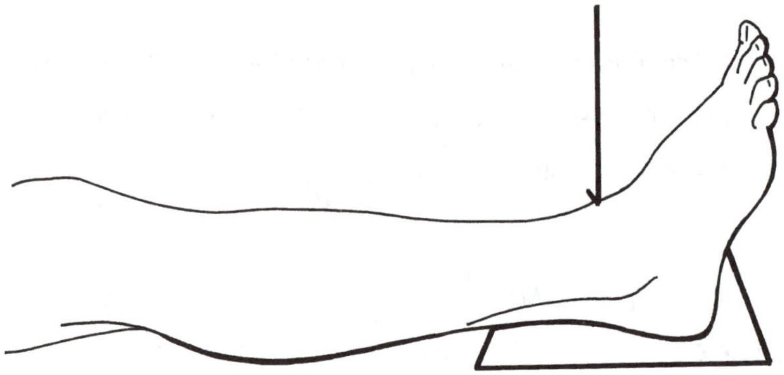

FIGURE 7–8. AP ankle.

NOTES

EVALUATOR SIGNATURE _____ DATE _____

► MEDIAL OBLIQUE ANKLE

OBJECTIVE: After practice, each student will position a patient for a medial oblique projection of the ankle.

PATIENT PREP: Remove the shoe and sock from the affected foot; roll the pant leg up.

FILM: 10 in. × 12 in. masked crosswise.

TASK ANALYSIS		CORRECTLY PERFORMED?	
MAJOR STEPS	KEY INFORMATION	YES	NO
1. Seat the patient on the table with the legs parallel to the long axis of the table.	The knee of the unaffected side can be flexed to relieve strain and make the patient more comfortable.		
2. Center the ankle joint to the unmasked half of the cassette.	The cassette may be positioned off-centered lengthwise to both the ankle joint and the central ray to include more of the distal lower leg.		
3. Dorsiflex the foot so the foot and leg are at a 90° angle.	This position may be very painful; move the patient slowly.		
4. Rotate the entire leg medially until the ankle and foot are inverted 15–20°.	The rotation should come from the hip and may, therefore, be rather uncomfortable. Support the hip with a sandbag, if necessary; immobilize the leg and foot with sandbags. An imaginary line between the two malleoli should be parallel with the film plane.		
5. Adjust the cassette so a point midway between the malleoli is centered to the unmasked half of the cassette.			
6. Direct the central ray perpendicular to the ankle joint.			
7. Collimate to include the proximal talus, medial and lateral malleoli, and distal fourth of the lower leg; use gonadal shielding.			

NOTE: *The distal tibiofibular joint can be demonstrated by internally rotating the leg and foot 45°. This may be the routine in some departments.*

CRITICAL ANATOMY: Mortise joint between distal tibia–fibula and proximal talus.

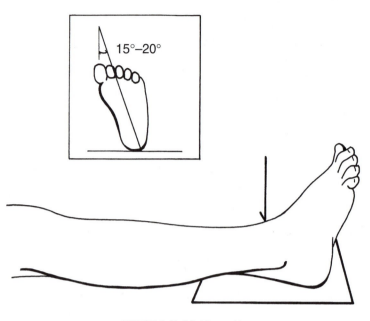

FIGURE 7–9. Medial oblique ankle.

NOTES

EVALUATOR SIGNATURE _____ DATE _____

► LATERAL ANKLE

OBJECTIVE: After practice, each student will position a patient for a lateral projection of the ankle.

PATIENT PREP: Remove the shoe and sock from the affected foot; roll the pant leg up.

FILM: 8 in. × 10 in. lengthwise or 9 in. × 9 in.

TASK ANALYSIS		CORRECTLY PERFORMED?	
MAJOR STEPS	KEY INFORMATION	YES	NO
1. Assist the patient to the lateral recumbent position on the table with the lateral surface of the affected ankle down.			
2. Adjust the cassette so the long axis is parallel to the lower leg.			
3. Center the ankle joint to the center of the cassette.	The cassette may be positioned off-centered lengthwise to both the ankle joint and the central ray to include more of the distal lower leg.		
4. With the foot dorsiflexed 90°, adjust the foot so the plantar surface is perpendicular to the film plane.	The lower leg should lie parallel with the film plane. If the knee is higher than the ankle, the cassette and foot should be elevated until the lower leg is parallel with the table-top.		
5. Direct the central ray perpendicular to the cassette through the center of the ankle joint.			
6. Collimate to include soft tissue of the distal fourth of lower leg and proximal talus; use gonadal shielding.			

NOTE: *On the finished radiograph, the distal fibula will be projected over the posterior portion of the tibia.*

CRITICAL ANATOMY: Posterior malleolus and tibiotalar joint.

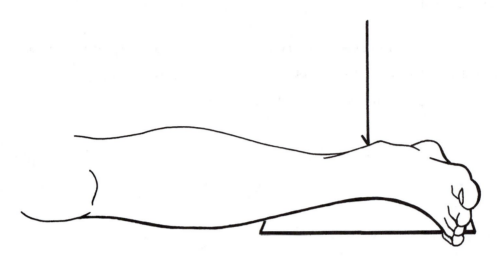

FIGURE 7–10. Lateral ankle.

NOTES
....

▶ AP LOWER LEG (TIBIA–FIBULA)

OBJECTIVE: After practice, each student will position a patient for an AP projection of the leg.

PATIENT PREP: Remove the shoe and sock from the affected foot; roll the pant leg up above the knee or gown the patient.

FILM: 7 in. × 17 in. lengthwise or 14 in. × 17 in. masked lengthwise, non-grid.

TASK ANALYSIS		CORRECTLY PERFORMED?	
MAJOR STEPS	KEY INFORMATION	YES	NO
1. Seat the patient on the table with the legs parallel to the long axis of the table.	The knee of the unaffected side can be flexed to relieve strain and make the patient more comfortable.		
2. Place the leg in anatomical position; dorsiflex the foot 90° and invert slightly.	The femoral epicondyles should be an equal distance from the cassette. Use sandbags to immobilize the foot, if necessary.		
3. Position the cassette so that points 1 to 1 1/2 in. beyond both the ankle and knee joints are included.	If the leg is longer than 17 in., position a 14 in. × 17 in. cassette diagonally (one projection per film) or include the ankle on the longer film and take separate AP and lateral knee projections on 10 in. × 12 in. cassettes.		
4. Direct the central ray perpendicular to the center of the lower leg and cassette.			
5. Collimate to soft tissue and at least 1 in. of the distal femur and proximal talus; use gonadal shielding.			

CRITICAL ANATOMY: Medial and lateral malleoli, tibial plateaus, intercondylar eminence, and shafts of the tibia and fibula.

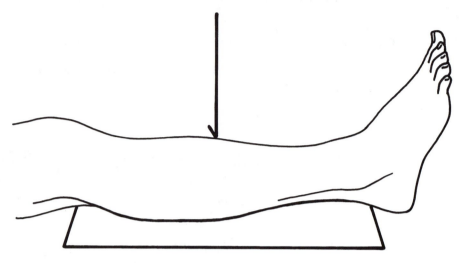

FIGURE 7–11. AP lower leg.

NOTES

EVALUATOR SIGNATURE _____ DATE _____

► LATERAL LOWER LEG (TIBIA–FIBULA)

OBJECTIVE: After practice, each student will position a patient for a lateral projection of the leg.

PATIENT PREP: Remove the shoe and sock from the affected foot; roll the pant leg up above the knee or gown the patient.

FILM: 7 in. × 17 in. lengthwise or 14 in. × 17 in. masked lengthwise, non-grid.

TASK ANALYSIS		CORRECTLY PERFORMED?	
MAJOR STEPS	KEY INFORMATION	YES	NO

1. Assist the patient to the lateral recumbent position on the table with the lateral surface of the affected ankle down.

2. Adjust the cassette so the long axis is parallel to the lower leg.

3. Dorsiflex the foot 90° and adjust the rotation of the body so the femoral epicondyles are superimposed (true lateral).

    The lower leg should lie parallel with the film plane. If the knee is higher, the ankle can be elevated using radiolucent supports.

4. Position the cassette so points 1 to 1 1/2 in. beyond both the ankle and knee joints are included.

    If the leg is longer than 17 in., position a 14 in. × 17 in. cassette diagonally (one projection per film) or include the ankle on the longer film and take separate AP and lateral knee projections on 10 in. × 12 in. cassettes.

5. Direct the central ray perpendicular to the center of the lower leg and cassette.

6. Collimate to soft tissue and at least 1 in. of the distal femur and proximal talus; use gonadal shielding.

CRITICAL ANATOMY: Tibial tuberosity, posterior malleolus, and shafts of the tibia and fibula.

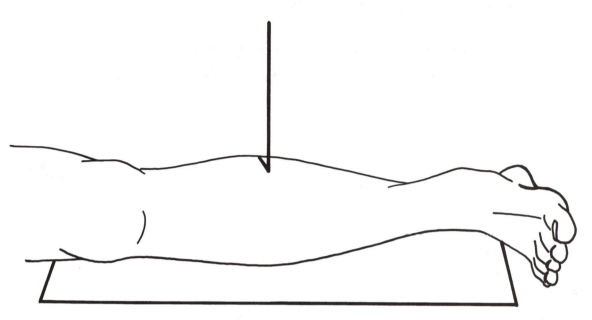

FIGURE 7–12. Lateral lower leg.

NOTES

▶ AP KNEE

OBJECTIVE: After practice, each student will position a patient for an AP projection of the knee.

PATIENT PREP: Roll the pant leg of the affected side up to mid-thigh or gown the patient; remove the shoe.

FILM: 10 in. × 12 in. or 8 in. × 10 in. lengthwise, grid or non-grid (depending on patient size and department routine).

TASK ANALYSIS		CORRECTLY PERFORMED?	
MAJOR STEPS	KEY INFORMATION	YES	NO
1. Seat the patient on the table with the affected leg extended and parallel to the long axis of the table.	The knee of the unaffected side can be flexed to relieve strain and make the patient more comfortable.		
2. Center the knee to the midline of the table or cassette.			
3. Adjust rotation of the leg so an imaginary line between the femoral epicondyles is parallel with the film plane.	Use sandbags to immobilize the leg, if necessary.		
4. Direct the central ray to enter at a point 1/2 in. below the apex of the patella: a. *Joint space:* 5–7° cephalad. b. *Distal femur and proximal lower leg:* Perpendicular.	The amount of central ray angle may depend on pathology or department policy.		
5. Center the cassette to the central ray.	The central ray should pass through the knee joint.		
6. Collimate to include soft tissue crosswise and to the film size lengthwise; use gonadal shielding.			

CRITICAL ANATOMY: Tibial plateaus, intercondylar eminence, medial and lateral condyles of the tibia, and medial and lateral condyles and epicondyles of the femur.

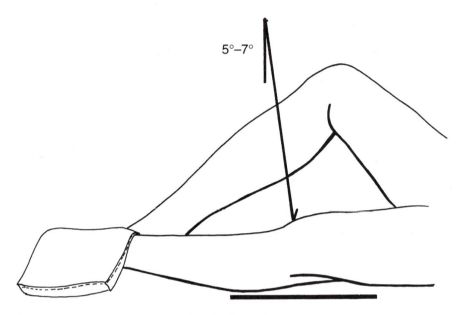

5°–7°

FIGURE 7–13. AP knee.

NOTES

► MEDIAL (INTERNAL) OBLIQUE KNEE

OBJECTIVE: After practice, each student will position a patient for a medial (internal) oblique projection of the knee.

PATIENT PREP: Roll the pant leg of the affected side up to mid-thigh or gown the patient; remove the shoe.

FILM: 10 in. × 12 in. or 8 in. × 10 in. lengthwise, grid or non-grid (depending on patient size and department routine).

TASK ANALYSIS		CORRECTLY PERFORMED?	
MAJOR STEPS	KEY INFORMATION	YES	NO
1. Seat the patient on the table with the affected leg extended and parallel to the long axis of the table.	The knee of the unaffected side can be flexed to relieve strain and make the patient more comfortable.		
2. Center the knee to the midline of the table or cassette.			
3. Rotate the entire leg 45° medially.	Palpate the femoral epicondyles to check positioning. It may be necessary to support the elevated hip with a sponge or sandbag; immobilize the leg with a sandbag, if necessary.		
4. Direct the central ray perpendicular or 5° cephalad to the knee joint at a point just distal to the level of the apex of the patella.			
5. Center the cassette to the central ray.			
6. Collimate to include soft tissue crosswise and to the film size lengthwise; use gonadal shielding.			

CRITICAL ANATOMY: Proximal tibiofibular articulation.

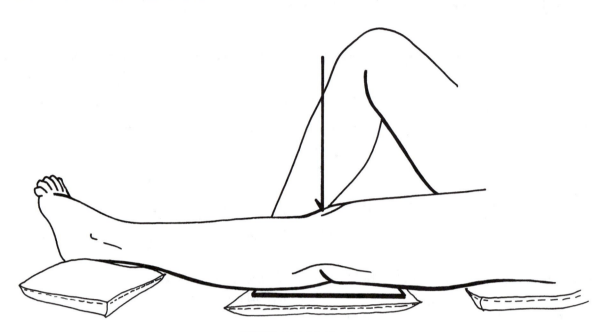

FIGURE 7–14. Medial oblique knee.

NOTES

► LATERAL (EXTERNAL) OBLIQUE KNEE

OBJECTIVE: After practice, each student will position a patient for a lateral (external) oblique projection of the knee.

PATIENT PREP: Roll the pant leg of the affected side up to mid-thigh or gown the patient; remove the shoe.

FILM: 10 in. × 12 in, or 8 in. × 10 in. lengthwise, grid or non-grid (depending on patient size and department routine).

TASK ANALYSIS		CORRECTLY PERFORMED?	
MAJOR STEPS	KEY INFORMATION	YES	NO
1. Seat the patient on the table with the affected leg extended and parallel to the long axis of the table.	The knee of the unaffected side can be flexed to relieve strain and make the patient more comfortable.		
2. Center the knee to the midline of the table or cassette.			
3. Rotate the entire leg 45° laterally.	Palpate the femoral epicondyles to check positioning. Immobilize the leg with a sandbag, if necessary.		
4. Direct the central ray perpendicular or 5° cephalad to the knee joint at a point just distal to the level of the apex of the patella.			
5. Center the cassette to the central ray.			
6. Collimate to include soft tissue crosswise and to the film size lengthwise; use gonadal shielding.			

CRITICAL ANATOMY: Tibia superimposed over the fibula.

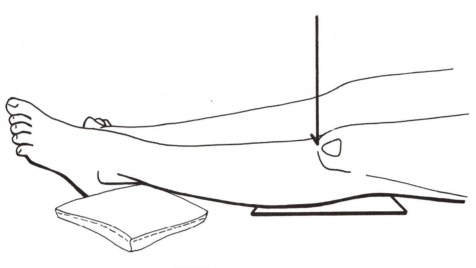

FIGURE 7–15. Lateral oblique knee.

NOTES
....

▶ LATERAL KNEE

OBJECTIVE: After practice, each student will position a patient for a lateral projection of the knee.

PATIENT PREP: Roll the pant leg of the affected side up to mid-thigh or gown the patient; remove the shoe.

FILM: 10 in. × 12 in. or 8 in. × 10 in. lengthwise, grid or non-grid (depending on patient size and department routine).

TASK ANALYSIS		CORRECTLY PERFORMED?	
MAJOR STEPS	KEY INFORMATION	YES	NO

1. Assist the patient to the lateral recumbent position on the table with the lateral surface of the affected knee down.

2. Center the femur to the midline of the table and flex the knee 20–30°.

3. Adjust the rotation of the leg so a line through the femoral epicondyles is perpendicular to the film plane.

   Flexing the knee of the unaffected leg and resting it on sponges or other support in front of the affected knee will help prevent overrotation.

4. Direct the central ray 5° cephalad to the knee joint.

   Angling the central ray prevents the joint space from being obscured by the magnified shadow of the medial femoral condyle. This can also be accomplished by elevating the ankle and lower leg with supports so the entire leg is parallel with the film plane.

5. Center the cassette to the central ray.

6. Collimate to include soft tissue crosswise and to the film size lengthwise; use gonadal shielding.

CRITICAL ANATOMY: Patella and tibial tuberosity.

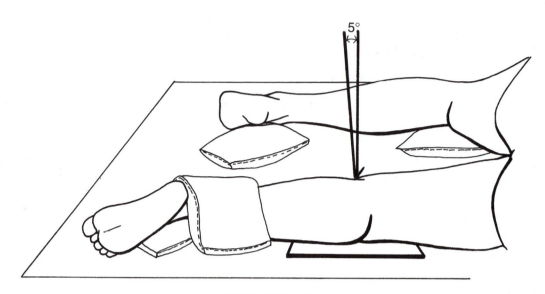

FIGURE 7–16. Lateral knee.

NOTES

....

► PA AXIAL INTERCONDYLAR FOSSA (CAMP–COVENTRY METHOD)

OBJECTIVE: After practice, each student will position a patient for a PA axial projection of the intercondylar fossa using the Camp–Coventry method.

PATIENT PREP: Roll the pant leg of the affected side up to mid-thigh or gown the patient; remove the shoe.

FILM: 8 in. × 10 in. crosswise or 9 in. × 9 in., non-grid.

TASK ANALYSIS		CORRECTLY PERFORMED?	
MAJOR STEPS	KEY INFORMATION	YES	NO
1. Assist the patient to the prone position with the affected leg parallel to the long axis of the table.	Adjust the body so there is no rotation; make sure the patient is relatively comfortable.		
2. Elevate both femurs using 2-in. sponges or other suitable supports.	Elevating both femurs prevents rotation and allows for easy placement of the cassette.		
3. Flex the knee so the lower leg forms an angle of approximately 40° with the table and rest the foot on a sponge or other support.	Adjust the leg so there is no medial or lateral rotation of the knee.		
4. Center the proximal half of the cassette to the knee joint and support the distal end with sandbags.	Although this projection can be obtained without angling the cassette, angling will reduce distortion of the intercondylar fossa.		
5. Direct the central ray through the knee joint and perpendicular to the long axis of the tibia.	The central ray should project the joint to the center of the film. If the lower leg forms a 40° angle with the table, the central ray should be directed 40° caudally.		
6. Collimate to include soft tissue crosswise and to the film size lengthwise; use gonadal shielding.			

CRITICAL ANATOMY: Intercondylar fossa.

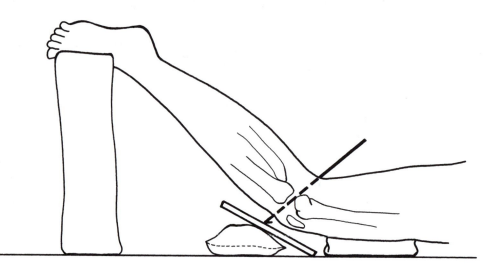

FIGURE 7–17. PA axial intercondylar fossa, Camp–Coventry method.

NOTES

▶ PA AXIAL INTERCONDYLAR FOSSA (HOLMBLAD METHOD)

OBJECTIVE: After practice, each student will position a patient for a PA axial projection of the intercondylar fossa using the Holmblad method.

PATIENT PREP: Roll the pant leg of the affected side up to mid-thigh or gown the patient; remove the shoe.

FILM: 8 in. × 10 in. crosswise or 9 in. × 9 in., non-grid or grid.

TASK ANALYSIS		CORRECTLY PERFORMED?	
MAJOR STEPS	KEY INFORMATION	YES	NO

1. Assist the patient to the kneeling position with the legs parallel to the long axis of the table.

   This position will be uncomfortable, so speed is important. If a grid is used, the leg must be centered to the midline of the grid.

2. Adjust the patient position so the angle between the femurs and table is approximately 70°.

   Check the foot and lower leg for rotation.

3. Direct the central ray perpendicular to the knee joint.

4. Center the cassette to the knee joint and central ray.

5. Collimate to include soft tissue crosswise and to the film size lengthwise; use gonadal shielding.

CRITICAL ANATOMY: Intercondylar fossa.

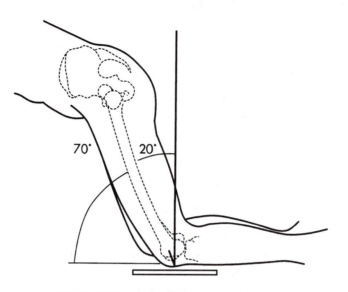

FIGURE 7–18. PA axial intercondylar fossa, Holmblad method.

NOTES
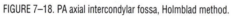

▶ AP AXIAL INTERCONDYLAR FOSSA (BECLERE METHOD)

OBJECTIVE: After practice, each student will position a patient for an AP axial projection of the intercondylar fossa using the Beclere method.

PATIENT PREP: Roll the pant leg of the affected side up to mid-thigh or gown the patient; remove the shoe.

FILM: 8 in. × 10 in. crosswise, 9 in. × 9 in., or curved cassette, non-grid.

TASK ANALYSIS		CORRECTLY PERFORMED?	
MAJOR STEPS	KEY INFORMATION	YES	NO
1. Assist the patient to the supine position with the affected leg parallel to the long axis of the table.	Adjust the leg so there is no rotation.		
2. Flex the affected knee to form a 120° angle between the long axes of the tibia and femur.	Move the patient slowly as flexion may be painful. Use sandbags or sponges to support the knee.		
3. Place the cassette under the knee so the center will coincide with the angled central ray.	Check for rotation and immobilize the foot with a sandbag.		
4. Direct the central ray perpendicular to the long axis of the tibia, centering to the knee joint.			
5. Collimate to include soft tissue crosswise and to the film size lengthwise; use gonadal shielding.			

CRITICAL ANATOMY: Intercondylar fossa.

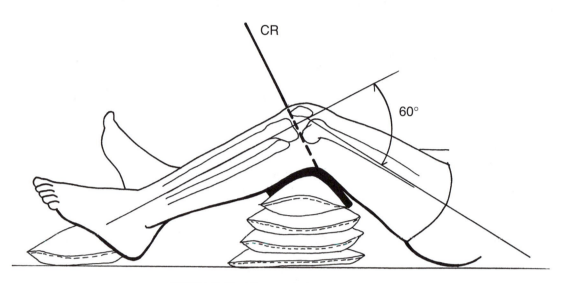

FIGURE 7–19. AP axial intercondylar fossa, Beclere method.

NOTES

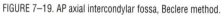

EVALUATOR SIGNATURE _____ DATE _____

► PA PATELLA

OBJECTIVE: After practice, each student will position a patient for a PA projection of the patella.

PATIENT PREP: Roll the pant leg of the affected side up to mid-thigh or gown the patient; remove the shoe.

FILM: 8 in. × 10 in. lengthwise or 9 in. × 9 in., grid or non-grid.

TASK ANALYSIS		CORRECTLY PERFORMED?	
MAJOR STEPS	KEY INFORMATION	YES	NO
1. Assist the patient to the prone position with the affected leg parallel to the long axis of the table.	Position supports under the feet to support the legs and relieve discomfort.		
2. Center the knee to the midline of the table or cassette.			
3. Rotate the heel 5–10° outward.			
4. Direct the central ray perpendicular to the patella.	The use of a cylinder cone (if available) will improve detail.		
5. Center the cassette to the central ray.			
6. Collimate to include soft tissue and 1 in. of the proximal tibia; use gonadal shielding.			

CRITICAL ANATOMY: Entire patella through the distal femur.

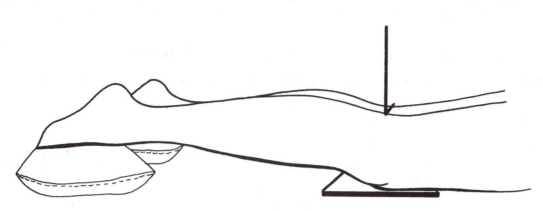

FIGURE 7–20. PA patella.

NOTES
....

► TANGENTIAL PATELLA & PATELLOFEMORAL JOINT ("SUNRISE," "SKYLINE," SETTEGAST METHOD)

OBJECTIVE: After practice, each student will position a patient for a tangential projection of the patella using the Settegast method.

PATIENT PREP: Roll the pant leg of the affected side up to mid-thigh or gown the patient; remove the shoe.

FILM: 8 in. × 10 in. crosswise or 9 in. × 9 in., non-grid.

TASK ANALYSIS		CORRECTLY PERFORMED?	
MAJOR STEPS	KEY INFORMATION	YES	NO
1. Assist the patient to the prone position with the affected leg parallel to the long axis of the table.	By maintaining the same part–film and tube–film relationships, this projection can also be performed with the patient in the supine or seated position.		
2. Set the technical factors.	This position may be very painful for the patient.		
3. Slowly flex the knee slightly more than 90°.	Wrap a strip of cloth, a belt, or other suitable device around the ankle and instruct the patient to hold the leg in position without letting it lean sideways. Too much flexion may make demonstration of the joint space difficult.		
4. Center the cassette under the patella.			
5. Direct the central ray to the joint space between the patella and the femoral condyles; the degree of angulation depends on the amount of knee flexion.	The central ray should be parallel to the long axis of the patella. Palpate the patella to determine its relationship with the film plane. The more the knee is bent, the less the central ray must be angled.		
6. Collimate to soft tissue, the distal femur, and the proximal lower leg; use gonadal shielding.	Recheck the centering to be sure the projected beam is centered to the film.		

NOTE: *This projection should not be attempted until a transverse fracture of the patella has been ruled out with a lateral projection.*

CRITICAL ANATOMY: Patella and patellofemoral joint space.

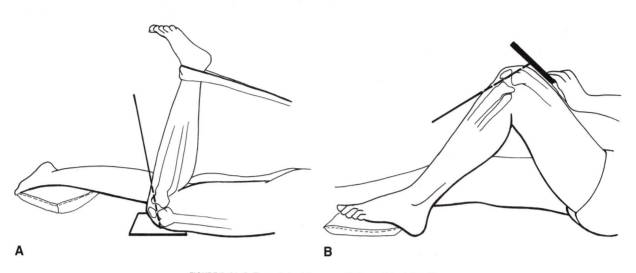

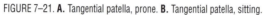

FIGURE 7–21. **A.** Tangential patella, prone. **B.** Tangential patella, sitting.

NOTES

▶ AP FEMUR

OBJECTIVE: After practice, each student will position a patient for an AP projection of the femur.

PATIENT PREP: Remove the pants and gown the patient; remove the shoe.

FILM: 7 in. × 17 in. or 14 in. × 17 in. lengthwise, and 10 in. × 12 in. lengthwise, grid.

TASK ANALYSIS		CORRECTLY PERFORMED?	
MAJOR STEPS	KEY INFORMATION	YES	NO
1. Assist the patient to the supine position with the affected leg parallel to the long axis of the table.	There should be no rotation of the body.		
2. Center the affected thigh to the midline of the table.	Move the unaffected leg away from the side of interest.		
3. Internally rotate the leg: a. 5° for the mid and distal femur. b. 15–20° for the proximal femur.	Inversion helps to compensate for the natural curvature of the femur. *If a fracture is suspected, do not invert the leg.*		
4. Take two projections to demonstrate the entire femur, including both joints: a. **Knee joint:** Place the lower border of the long cassette 2 in. below the knee joint. b. **Hip joint:** Center the 10 in. × 12 in. cassette to the level of the greater trochanter.	The greater trochanter is palpable on the proximal lateral aspect of the femur.		
5. Direct the central ray perpendicular to the center of the cassette.			
6. Collimate to include soft tissue and 1 to 2 in. beyond the joint; use gonadal shielding.			

CRITICAL ANATOMY: Femoral condyles and epicondyles, greater trochanter, femoral neck, femoral head, and femoral shaft.

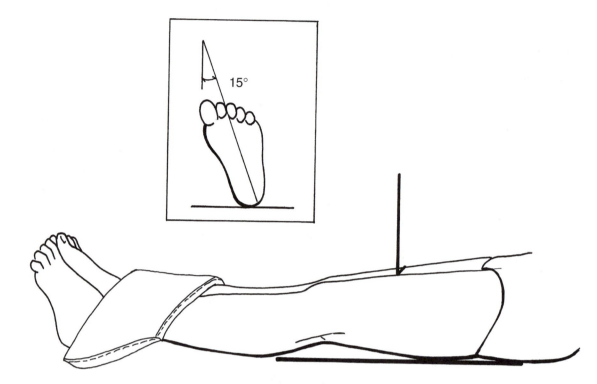

FIGURE 7–22. AP femur.

NOTES

EVALUATOR SIGNATURE _____ DATE _____

► LATERAL FEMUR

OBJECTIVE: After practice, each student will position a patient for a lateral projection of the femur.

PATIENT PREP: Remove the pants and gown the patient; remove the shoe.

FILM: 7 in. × 17 in. or 14 in. × 17 in. lengthwise, and 10 in. × 12 in. lengthwise, grid.

TASK ANALYSIS		CORRECTLY PERFORMED?	
MAJOR STEPS	KEY INFORMATION	YES	NO

MAJOR STEPS	KEY INFORMATION	YES	NO
1. Assist the patient to the lateral recumbent position with the affected side down.	*If a fracture is suspected, do* not *move the patient;* use a horizontal central ray for a cross-table lateral projection.		
2. Center the affected thigh to the midline of the table.	Adjust the leg so it is parallel to the long axis of the table.		
3. Take two projections to demonstrate the entire femur, including both joints:			
a. ***Knee joint:*** Bring the unaffected extremity in front of the affected side, keeping the pelvis in a true lateral position. Adjust rotation of the body and leg so an imaginary line through the femoral epicondyles is perpendicular to the film. Place the lower border of the longer cassette 2 in. below the knee joint.	Support the unaffected leg with sponges or pillows to immobilize and prevent rotation of the pelvis.		
b. ***Hip joint:*** Draw the unaffected leg behind the affected side and rotate the pelvis backward 10–15° from lateral; place the upper border of the small cassette 2 in. above the hip joint.	Estimate the location of the hip joint by the bend of the leg.		
4. Direct the central ray perpendicular to the center of the cassette.			
5. Collimate to include soft tissue and 1 to 2 in. beyond the joint; use gonadal shielding.			

CRITICAL ANATOMY: Femoral condyles superimposed, lesser trochanter, femoral head, femoral neck, and femoral shaft.

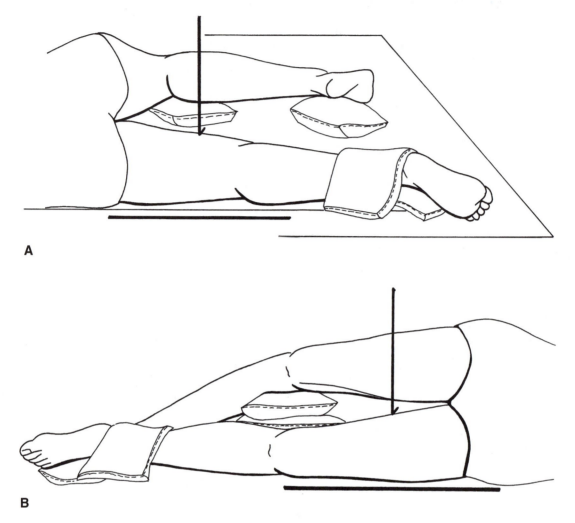

A

B

FIGURE 7–23. **A.** Distal femur, lateral position. **B.** Proximal femur, lateral position using a 14 in. × 17 in. cassette.

NOTES

....

PELVIC GIRDLE

► AP PELVIS

OBJECTIVE: After practice, each student will position a patient for an AP projection of the pelvis.

PATIENT PREP: Remove all clothing below the waist except the socks; gown the patient.

FILM: 14 in. × 17 in. crosswise, grid.

TASK ANALYSIS		CORRECTLY PERFORMED?	
MAJOR STEPS	KEY INFORMATION	YES	NO
1. Position the patient supine on the table.			
2. Center the median plane of the body to the midline of the table.	Align the patient to the long axis of the table.		
3. Adjust the body to true AP position with no rotation by palpating the anterior superior iliac spines (ASISs) and positioning them equidistant from the tabletop.	Very thin or injured patients may need support with sponges.		
4. Grasp the patient's heels and rotate the legs internally until the longitudinal planes of the feet are inverted 15–20°.	Immobilize with sandbags, tape, etc. *If a fracture is suspected, do not invert the legs.*		
5. Put the upper border of the cassette 2 in. above the iliac crests.	Adjust centering as needed to place the pelvis in the center of the film.		
6. Direct the central ray perpendicular to the center of the cassette.			
7. Collimate to include the femoral trochanters and iliac crests crosswise and lengthwise.			
8. Make the exposure during suspended *expiration.*			

NOTE: *Externally rotate the legs to demonstrate the lesser trochanters.*

CRITICAL ANATOMY: Iliac crests, alae, ASISs, ischia, pubic bones, symphysis pubis, acetabula, femoral heads and necks, and greater trochanters.

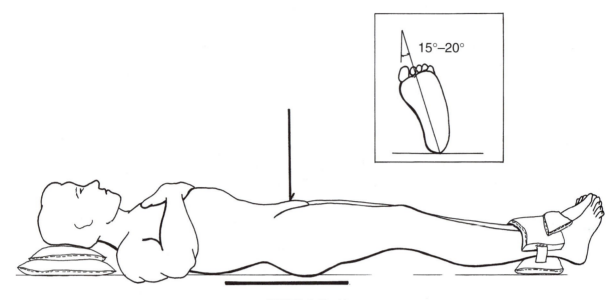

FIGURE 8–1. AP pelvis.

NOTES
....

EVALUATOR SIGNATURE _____ DATE _____

▶ AP HIP

OBJECTIVE: After practice, each student will position a patient for an AP projection of the hip.

PATIENT PREP: Remove all clothing below the waist except the socks; gown the patient.

FILM: 10 in. × 12 in. lengthwise, grid.

TASK ANALYSIS		CORRECTLY PERFORMED?	
MAJOR STEPS	KEY INFORMATION	YES	NO

1. Position the patient supine on the table.

2. Center the sagittal plane passing 2 in. medial to the ASIS to the midline of the table.

   Align the patient to the long axis of the table.

3. Invert the leg 15–20° by grasping the heel of the foot and turning the leg medially.

   If a fracture is suspected, do not invert the leg. Immobilize with a sandbag.

4. Direct the central ray perpendicular to the level of the highest point of the greater trochanter.

   When the leg is inverted, the greater trochanter is readily palpable on the lateral aspect of the proximal femur.

5. Center the cassette to the central ray.

6. Collimate to include the ASIS and the femoral trochanters crosswise and lengthwise; use gonadal shielding.

7. Make the exposure during suspended *expiration.*

NOTE: *For the initial hip examination, the AP projection of the entire pelvis is usually obtained. Follow-up studies may include only the affected side.*

CRITICAL ANATOMY: Greater trochanter, femoral head and neck, and acetabulum.

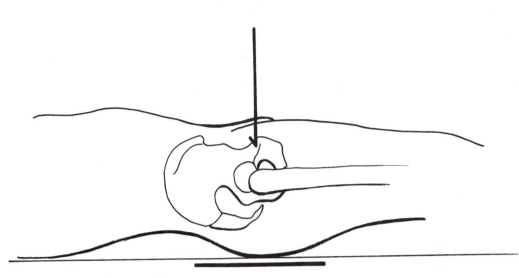

FIGURE 8–2. AP hip.

NOTES
....

▶ AP OBLIQUE HIP (MODIFIED CLEAVES METHOD— "FROG-LEG" LATERAL)

OBJECTIVE: After practice, each student will position a patient for an AP oblique projection of the hip in the "frog-leg" position.

PATIENT PREP: Remove all clothing below the waist except the socks; gown the patient and drape with a sheet.

FILM: 10 in. × 12 in. crosswise, grid.

TASK ANALYSIS		CORRECTLY PERFORMED?	
MAJOR STEPS	KEY INFORMATION	YES	NO

MAJOR STEPS	KEY INFORMATION	YES	NO
1. Position the patient supine on the table.	Align the patient to the long axis of the table.		
2. Center the sagittal plane passing through the ASIS to the midline of the table.			
3. Flex the knee and hip of the affected side until the foot reaches the knee of the opposite leg.	Move the patient slowly since this position may be somewhat painful.		
4. Abduct the flexed extremity 40°.	Immobilize the foot with a sandbag; pillows may be used to support the knee.		
5. Direct the central ray perpendicular to the hip joint.	The central ray will enter approximately at the bend in the hip.		
6. Center the cassette to the central ray.			
7. Collimate to include the acetabulum and the proximal third of the femur; use gonadal shielding.			
8. Make the exposure during suspended *expiration*.			

NOTE: *To better demonstrate the femoral necks, angle the tube to direct the central ray parallel to the long axis of the femur.*

CRITICAL ANATOMY: Lesser trochanter, femoral head, acetabulum, and proximal femur.

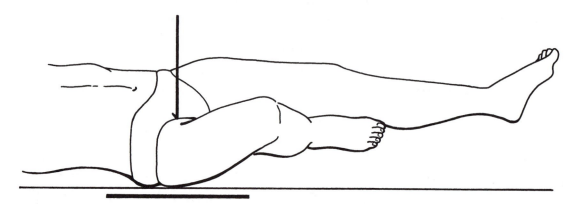

FIGURE 8–3. AP oblique hip (modified Cleaves method—"frog-leg" lateral).

NOTES
....

▶ LATERAL HIP (LAUENSTEIN METHOD)

OBJECTIVE: After practice, each student will position a patient for a lateral projection of the hip using the Lauenstein method.

PATIENT PREP: Remove all clothing below the waist except the socks; gown the patient and drape with a sheet.

FILM: 10 in. × 12 in. crosswise, grid.

TASK ANALYSIS		CORRECTLY PERFORMED?	
MAJOR STEPS	KEY INFORMATION	YES	NO
1. Rotate the patient from the supine position toward the affected side, resting the femur against the table.	The patient's body will be positioned obliquely and the femur will be in a lateral position.		
2. Center the affected hip to the midline of the table.			
3. Flex the knee and hip of the affected side and draw the thigh up to near-90° angle position.	Extend the opposite thigh and support the hip with sponges.		
4. Adjust the position of the pelvis so the upper side is rotated posteriorly enough to prevent superimposition on the affected hip.			
5. Direct the central ray perpendicular to a point midway between the ASIS and the pubic symphysis.	This projection will demonstrate the relationship of the femoral head to the acetabulum.		
6. Center the cassette to the central ray.			
7. Collimate to include the acetabulum and the proximal third of the femur; use gonadal shielding, if possible.			
8. Make the exposure during suspended *expiration.*			

NOTE: *This position is not used when there is an unhealed fracture or destructive disease due to the danger of fragment displacement or injury.*

CRITICAL ANATOMY: Femoral head, acetabulum, and proximal femur.

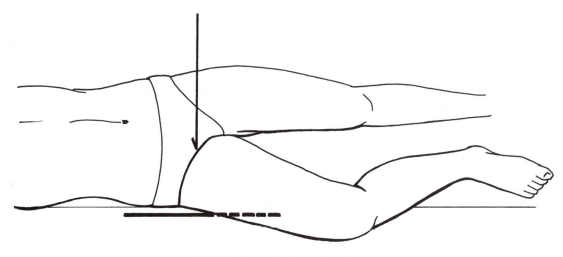

FIGURE 8–4. Lateral hip (Lauenstein method).

NOTES
....

► TRANSFEMORAL (SURGICAL, CROSS-TABLE) LATERAL HIP

OBJECTIVE: After practice, each student will position a patient for a transfemoral lateral projection of the hip.

PATIENT PREP: Remove all clothing below the waist except the socks; gown the patient and drape with a sheet.

FILM: 10 in. × 12 in. lengthwise, grid.

TASK ANALYSIS		CORRECTLY PERFORMED?	
MAJOR STEPS	KEY INFORMATION	YES	NO
1. Position the patient supine on the table. 2. Elevate the affected hip with a sponge.	Align the patient to the long axis of the table.		
3. Support the cassette in the vertical position next to the affected hip with the side nearest the patient's head at the iliac crest; angle the opposite end away from the patient until the cassette is parallel to the femoral neck.	The axis of the femoral neck can be identified by bisected an imaginary line between the ASIS and the pubic symphysis and drawing a perpendicular line from that point.		
4. Flex the knee and hip of the unaffected side and elevate the leg.	Flexion and elevation should remove the unaffected leg from the path of the central ray; support under the foot will be needed.		
5. Invert the leg of the affected side 15–20° and immobilize.	*Do not invert the leg if there is a possibility of a fracture.*		
6. Direct the central ray horizontally and perpendicular to the femoral neck and the center of the cassette.	If the position of the cassette is correct, the central ray will be perpendicular to it. Maintain a 40-in. SID.		
7. Collimate to include the acetabulum, proximal third of the femur, and ischial tuberosity.			
8. Make the exposure during suspended respiration.			

CRITICAL ANATOMY: Femoral head, acetabulum, and proximal femur.

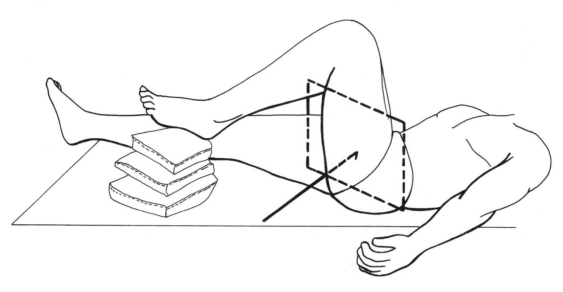

FIGURE 8–5. Transfemoral lateral hip.

NOTES

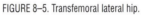

▶ AP OBLIQUE SACROILIAC JOINTS

OBJECTIVE: After practice, each student will position a patient for both AP oblique projections of the sacroiliac joints.

PATIENT PREP: Remove all clothing below the waist except shoes and socks; gown the patient.

FILM: 8 in. × 10 in. lengthwise, 9 in. × 9 in. or 10 in. × 12 in. crosswise, grid.

TASK ANALYSIS		CORRECTLY PERFORMED?	
MAJOR STEPS	KEY INFORMATION	YES	NO
1. Position the patient supine on the table.	Align the patient to the long axis of the table.		
2. Rotate the patient to the 25–30° RPO or LPO position, elevating the side being examined.	The entire body should be rotated the same amount; use sponges for support. The patient may reach across the body and grasp the side of the table; the knees should be slightly flexed.		
3. Center the patient so that the sagittal plane 1 in. medial to the elevated ASIS is centered to the table.	The joint furthest from the table will be demonstrated.		
4. Direct the central ray perpendicular to the center of the cassette through a point 1 in. medial to the ASIS.			
5. Center the cassette to the central ray.			
6. Collimate to include the elevated sacroiliac joint; use gonadal shielding, if possible.			
7. Make the exposure during suspended respiration.			
8. Examine the opposite side in the same manner.	Both sides must be examined for comparison.		

CRITICAL ANATOMY: Sacroiliac joint furthest from the film.

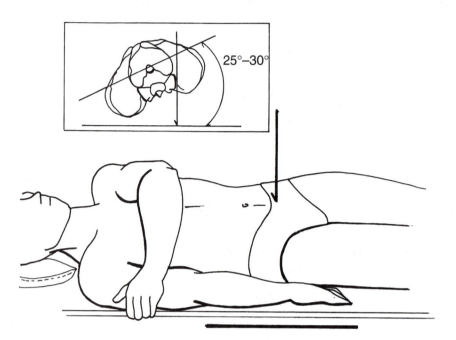

FIGURE 8–6. RPO, left sacroiliac joint.

NOTES

▶ AP AXIAL ANTERIOR PELVIC BONES (TAYLOR METHOD) (OUTLET)

OBJECTIVE: After practice, each student will correctly position a patient to demonstrate the anterior pelvic bones using the Taylor method.

PATIENT PREP: Remove all clothing below the waist except shoes and socks; gown the patient.

FILM: 11 in. × 14 in. or 10 in. × 12 in. crosswise (anterior pelvic bones only); 14 in. × 17 in. (entire outlet), grid.

TASK ANALYSIS		CORRECTLY PERFORMED?	
MAJOR STEPS	KEY INFORMATION	YES	NO

MAJOR STEPS	KEY INFORMATION
1. Position the patient supine on the table.	Align the body to the long axis of the table.
2. Center the midsagittal plane of the body to the midline of the table and adjust to true AP position.	The ASISs should be equal distance from the table.
3. Direct the central ray: a. *Females:* 30–45° cephalad to a point 2 in. distal to the upper border of the symphysis pubis. b. *Males:* 20–35° cephalad to a point 2 in. distal to the upper border of the symphysis pubis.	This centering point may be localized accurately by palpating the lateral aspect of the greater trochanter. To include the entire pelvic outlet on a 14 in. × 17 in. film, centering should be slightly higher.
4. Center the cassette to the central ray.	
5. Collimate to include the ASISs and ischial tuberosities crosswise and lengthwise.	
6. Make exposure during suspended respiration.	

CRITICAL ANATOMY: Pubic and ischial rami, symphysis pubis, ischial tuberosities, and obturator foramina.

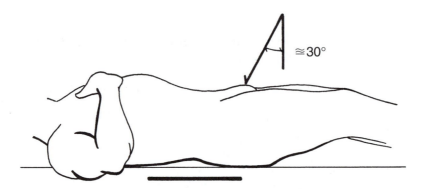

FIGURE 8–7. AP axial anterior pelvic bones (Taylor method).

NOTES
....

► SUPEROINFERIOR AXIAL ANTERIOR PELVIC BONES (LILIENFELD METHOD) (INLET)

OBJECTIVE: After practice, each student will correctly position a patient to demonstrate the anterior pelvic bones using the Lilienfeld method.

PATIENT PREP: Remove all clothing below the waist except shoes and socks; gown the patient.

FILM: 11 in. × 14 in. or 10 in. × 12 in. crosswise (anterior pelvic bones only); 14 in. × 17 in. (entire inlet), grid.

TASK ANALYSIS		CORRECTLY PERFORMED?	
MAJOR STEPS	KEY INFORMATION	YES	NO
1. Assist the patient to the seated erect position on the table.	The legs should be extended and the body should be parallel to the long axis of the table.		
2. Center the midsagittal plane to the midline of the table.	To relieve strain, flex the knees slightly and support with sponges or a pillow.		
3. Instruct the patient to lean backwards 45–50°, using the arms for support; the back should be arched to place the pubic arch in a vertical position.	The patient will be in a semi-sitting position.		
4. Direct the central ray perpendicular to a point 1 1/2 in. superior to the symphysis pubis (anterior pelvic bones or pelvic inlet, respectively).	Centering should be slightly higher when imaging the pelvic inlet.		
5. Center the cassette to the central ray.			
6. Collimate to the hip joints and ischial tuberosities (anterior pelvic bones).			
7. Make the exposure during suspended respiration.			

NOTE: *This projection may also be obtained by positioning the patient supine and directing the central ray 35–45° caudally.*

CRITICAL ANATOMY: Bodies and rami of ishia and pubic bones, ischial tuberosities, and symphysis pubis.

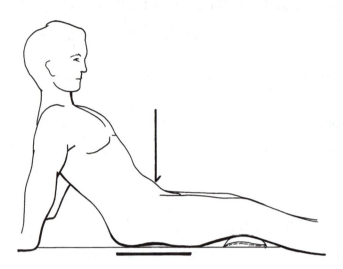

FIGURE 8–8. Superoinferior axial anterior pelvic bones (Lilienfeld method).

NOTES
....

BONY THORAX

▶ AP RIBS: ABOVE & BELOW THE DIAPHRAGM

OBJECTIVE: After practice, each student will position a patient for an AP projection of the ribs, above and below the diaphragm.

PATIENT PREP: Remove all clothing and jewelry above the hips; gown the patient.

FILM: 14 in. × 17 in. crosswise or lengthwise, grid.

TASK ANALYSIS		CORRECTLY PERFORMED?	
MAJOR STEPS	KEY INFORMATION	YES	NO
1. Position the patient supine with the body parallel to the long axis of the table.	Check for rotation. This examination may be performed with the patient erect; a PA projection may be obtained if the area of interest is in the anterior ribs.		
2. Determine the exact location of the lesion.	Ask the patient to point to the area of pain.		
3. Center the median plane (bilateral study) or sagittal plane midway between the spine and lateral margin of the thorax (unilateral study) to the midline of the table.			
4. Ribs above the diaphragm:			
a. Position the cassette so the upper border is 2 in. above the top of the shoulders.			
b. Direct the central ray perpendicular to the midpoint of the cassette.			
c. Collimate to include the lateral ribs and C-7; use gonadal shielding.			
d. Make the exposure during suspended deep *inspiration.*	Breathing may by painful so allow time for the patient to breathe slowly.		
5. Ribs below the diaphragm:			
a. Position the cassette so the lower border is 1 1/2 in. below the iliac crests.	Approximately 1/2 in. of the crests should be seen on the finished radiograph. Make sure there will be at least 1 to 2 in. of overlap on the finished radiographs.		
b. Direct the central ray perpendicular to the midpoint of the cassette.			
c. Collimate to include the lateral ribs and iliac crests; use gonadal shielding.			
d. Make the exposure during suspended *expiration.*			

CRITICAL ANATOMY: Anterior and posterior aspects of the ribs.

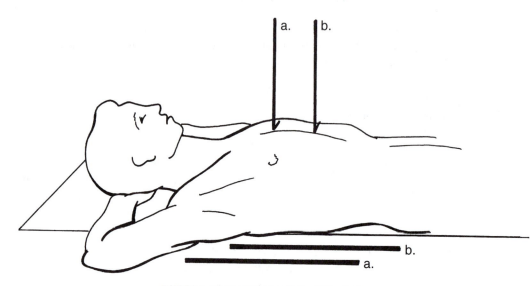

FIGURE 9–1. AP ribs above (a) and below (b) the diaphragm.

NOTES
....

.

▶ AP OBLIQUE (RPO & LPO) RIBS: ABOVE & BELOW THE DIAPHRAGM

OBJECTIVE: After practice, each student will position a patient for AP oblique projections of the ribs, above and below the diaphragm.

PATIENT PREP: Remove all clothing and jewelry above the waist; gown the patient.

FILM: 14 in. × 17 in. lengthwise, grid.

TASK ANALYSIS		CORRECTLY PERFORMED?	
MAJOR STEPS	KEY INFORMATION	YES	NO
1. Position the patient supine with the body parallel to the long axis of the table.	This examination may be performed with the patient erect; PA oblique projections may be obtained if the area of interest is in the anterior ribs.		
2. Determine the exact location of the lesion.	Ask the patient to point to the area of pain.		
3. Rotate the patient 45° toward the affected side.	Use sponges to support and immobilize the patient.		
4. Center the plane halfway between the spine and the lateral surface of the thorax to the midline of the table.			
5. Raise the arm of the dependent side (side down) above the head and rest it on the table.	Abducting the arm pulls the scapula away from the rib cage.		
6. Ribs above the diaphragm: a. Position the cassette so the upper border is 2 in. above the top of the shoulders. b. Direct the central ray perpendicular to the the midpoint of the cassette. c. Collimate to include the lateral ribs and C-7; use gonadal shielding. d. Make exposure during suspended deep *inspiration.*			
7. Ribs below the diaphragm: a. Position the cassette so the lower border is 1 1/2 in. below the iliac crests. b. Direct the central ray perpendicular to the midpoint of the cassette.	Make sure there will be at least 2 in. of overlap on the finished radiographs.		

Continued

TASK ANALYSIS		CORRECTLY PERFORMED?	
MAJOR STEPS	KEY INFORMATION	YES	NO

c. Collimate to include the lateral ribs and iliac crests; use gonadal shielding.

d. Make exposure during suspended *expiration.*

CRITICAL ANATOMY: Axillary ribs of the side nearest the film; vertebral ends of the ribs furthest from the film.

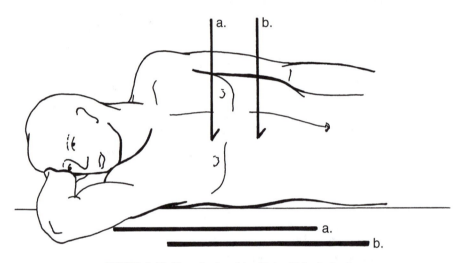

FIGURE 9–2. AP oblique ribs above (a) and below (b) the diaphragm.

NOTES

EVALUATOR SIGNATURE _____   DATE _____

▶ RAO STERNUM

OBJECTIVE: After practice, each student will position a patient for an RAO projection of the sternum.

PATIENT PREP: Remove all clothing and jewelry above the waist; gown the patient.

FILM: 10 in. × 12 in. lengthwise, grid.

TASK ANALYSIS		CORRECTLY PERFORMED?	
MAJOR STEPS	KEY INFORMATION	YES	NO

MAJOR STEPS	KEY INFORMATION
1. Assist the patient to the RAO position on the table.	
2. Adjust the body to a 15–20° angle between the anterior surface of the body and the table top.	The degree of obliquity will vary with the thickness of the patient; thin patients must be rotated more than deep-chested patients. Rotate only enough to prevent superimposition of the spine and sternum.
3. Center the cassette to the midsternal area.	The upper border of the cassette will approximately be at the level of the spinous process of C-7.
4. Direct the central ray perpendicular to the center of the cassette.	
5. Collimate to the include the sternal ends of the clavicles and xiphoid process; use gonadal shielding.	
6. Breathing instructions may be either: a. *Quiet breathing,* or b. Suspended *expiration.*	Breathing motion will obliterate the pulmonary markings.

CRITICAL ANATOMY: Manubrium, body and xiphoid process of the sternum, and right sternoclavicular joint.

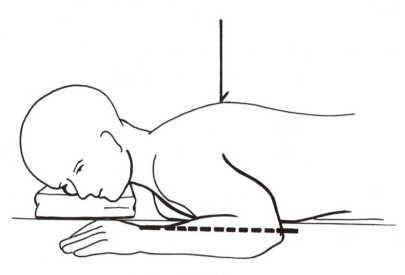

FIGURE 9–3. RAO sternum.

NOTES

► LATERAL STERNUM

OBJECTIVE: After practice, each student will position a patient for a lateral projection of the sternum.

PATIENT PREP: Remove all clothing and jewelry above the waist; gown the patient.

FILM: 10 in. × 12 in. lengthwise, grid.

TASK ANALYSIS		CORRECTLY PERFORMED?	
MAJOR STEPS	KEY INFORMATION	YES	NO
1. Assist the patient to the lateral erect position in front of the upright grid device.	The patient may be sitting or standing.		
2. Rotate the shoulders back and place the patient's hands behind the back.			
3. Center the sternum to the midline of the upright grid device.	Keep the sagittal plane of the body vertical.		
4. Center the cassette to the sternum.	Palpate the manubrial notch and the xiphoid process to assist in centering. When centered, the upper border of the cassette should be approximately 1 1/2 in. above the manubrial notch.		
5. Adjust the patient so the plane of the sternum is at a right angle to the film plane.	The broad surface of the sternum should be perpendicular to the cassette.		
6. Direct the central ray perpendicular (horizontally) to the center of the cassette using 72-in. SID.			
7. Collimate to include the manubrium and xiphoid process; use gonadal shielding.			
8. Make the exposure during suspended deep *inspiration*.	Deep inspiration moves the sternum anterior to the ribs and provides sharper contrast between the posterior surface of the sternum and the adjacent structures.		

NOTE: *In cases of severe injury, the patient can be examined in the supine position using a horizontal central ray. This recumbent position is also recommended for radiographing large-breasted women.*

CRITICAL ANATOMY: Manubrium, body, xiphoid process, and sternal angle.

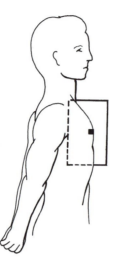

FIGURE 9–4. Lateral sternum.

NOTES
....

▶ PA OBLIQUE STERNOCLAVICULAR JOINTS

OBJECTIVE: After practice, each student will position a patient for RAO and LAO projections of the sternoclavicular joints.

PATIENT PREP: Remove all clothing and jewelry above the waist; gown the patient.

FILM: 8 in. × 10 in. crosswise or 9 in. × 9 in., grid.

TASK ANALYSIS		CORRECTLY PERFORMED?	
MAJOR STEPS	KEY INFORMATION	YES	NO
1. Position the patient prone with the body parallel to the long axis of the table.	The arm of the side of interest should be alongside the patient.		
2. Assist the patient into a shallow oblique position (approximately 10–15°).	Rotate the patient only enough to project the vertebral shadow well behind the sternoclavicular joint. This will vary with the thickness of the patient; thinner patients will need to be turned more than larger patients. The patient can bend the arm and leg of the opposite side to support the body.		
3. Center the joint to the midline of the table.			
4. Center the cassette to the level of the sternoclavicular joint.			
5. Direct the central ray perpendicular to the midpoint of the cassette.			
6. Collimate to include the sternal ends of the clavicles and the manubrium; use gonadal shielding.			
7. Make the exposure during suspended *expiration*.			

NOTE: *Both joints are usually examined for comparison.*

CRITICAL ANATOMY: Sternoclavicular joint nearest the table.

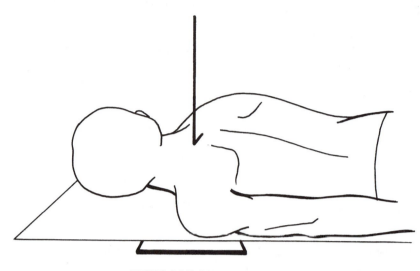

FIGURE 9–5. LAO (left) sternoclavicular joint.

NOTES
....

VERTEBRAL COLUMN

10

► AP CERVICAL SPINE

OBJECTIVE: After practice, each student will position a patient for an AP projection of the cervical spine.

PATIENT PREP: Remove hairpins, dental appliances, earrings, necklaces, glasses, and bra; gown the patient.

FILM: 10 in. × 12 in. or 8 in. × 10 in. lengthwise, grid.

TASK ANALYSIS		CORRECTLY PERFORMED?	
MAJOR STEPS	KEY INFORMATION	YES	NO
1. Assist the patient to the supine position on the table.	The patient may flex the knees and hips to place the plantar surface of feet on the table for comfort. The projection may also be obtained with the patient sitting or standing in front of an upright grid device.		
2. Center the midsagittal plane to the midline of the table; pull gently on the patient's legs or under the patient's arms to straighten.	Make sure the head and shoulders are not rotated.		
3. Extend the patient's head so that a line between the occlusal plane and the mastoid tips is perpendicular to the film plane.	This positioning should prevent superimposition of the mandible and the midcervical vertebrae.		
4. Direct the central ray through C-4 at an angle of 15–20° cephalad.	The central ray should enter at or slightly inferior to the most prominent point of the thyroid cartilage. The degree of angulation depends on the amount of cervical spine curvature.		
5. Center the cassette to the central ray.	The top of the cassette should be approximately at the top of the patient's ear.		
6. Collimate to the neck crosswise and to the film lengthwise; use gonadal shielding.			
7. Make the exposure during suspended respiration.			

CRITICAL ANATOMY: Lower five cervical bodies, interpediculate spaces, transverse processes, and intervertebral disk spaces.

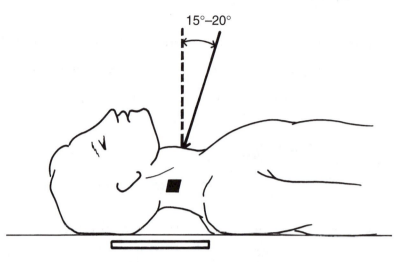

FIGURE 10–1. AP cervical spine.

NOTES

▶ AP ATLAS AND AXIS (OPEN-MOUTH ODONTOID)

OBJECTIVE: After practice, each student will position a patient for an AP open-mouth projection of the 1st and 2nd cervical vertebrae.

PATIENT PREP: Remove hairpins, dental appliances, earrings, necklaces, glasses, and bra; gown the patient.

FILM: 8 in. × 10 in. lengthwise or 9 in. × 9 in., grid.

TASK ANALYSIS		CORRECTLY PERFORMED?	
MAJOR STEPS	KEY INFORMATION	YES	NO
1. Assist the patient to the supine position on the table.	The patient may flex the knees and hips to place the plantar surface of feet on the table for comfort. The projection may also be obtained with the patient sitting or standing in front of an upright grid device.		
2. Adjust the patient's head and body so the midsagittal plane is centered to and parallel with the long axis of the table.			
3. Set the technical factors.	The patient position may be difficult to maintain; be prepared.		
4. Instruct the patient to open the mouth as wide as possible.	The head may have to be elevated slightly with a small sponge.		
5. Position the head so a line from the lower margin of the upper incisors to the level of the tips of the mastoid processes is perpendicular to the film.	If the patient has a broad head or long mandible, the entire atlas will not be demonstrated. When the exactly superimposed shadows of the inferior margins of the upper teeth and base of the skull are in line with the mastoid tips, the position cannot be improved.		
6. Direct the central ray perpendicular to C-1 through the midpoint of the open mouth.	A 30- to 32-in. SID can be used to magnify the open mouth for better visualization of the atlas and axis.		
7. Center the cassette to the central ray.			
8. Collimate to a 5 in. × 5 in. field size; use gonadal shielding.	Be sure to include marker in the collimation field.		
9. Direct the patient to open the mouth wide and softly say "ah" during the exposure.	Phonation will hold the tongue on the floor of the mouth so the shadow will not be projected on the atlas and the axis; this action will also immobilize the mandible.		

CRITICAL ANATOMY: Atlas (C-1), axis (C-2), dens, transverse processes of C-1, zygapophyseal joints between C-1 and C-2, and intervertebral disk space between C-1 and C-2.

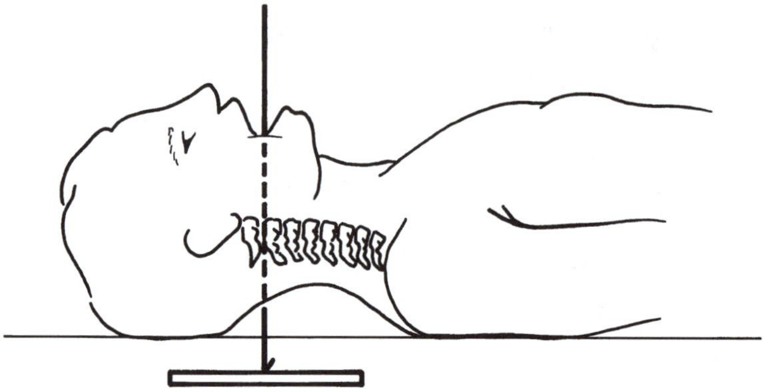

FIGURE 10–2. AP atlas and axis.

NOTES

EVALUATOR SIGNATURE _____   DATE _____

▶ AP AXIAL OBLIQUE CERVICAL SPINE

OBJECTIVE: After practice, each student will position a patient for AP axial oblique projection of the cervical spine.

PATIENT PREP: Remove hairpins, dental appliances, earrings, necklaces, glasses, and bra; gown the patient.

FILM: 10 in. × 12 in. or 8 in. × 10 in. lengthwise, grid or non-grid.

TASK ANALYSIS		CORRECTLY PERFORMED?	
MAJOR STEPS	KEY INFORMATION	YES	NO

1. Assist the patient to the AP erect position in front of the upright grid device.	The patient may be sitting or standing. The projection may also be obtained with the patient recumbent on the table.		
2. Rotate the entire body and head to form a 45° angle between the coronal plane and the film plane.	The adjacent shoulder should be placed firmly against the upright grid device for support. Check the degree of rotation with a protractor.		
3. Center the cervical spine to the midline of the upright grid device.			
4. Turn the head away from the side being examined (the side furthest from the film).	Be careful not to rotate the spine. Turn the head just enough to prevent superimposition of the mandibular rami and the intervertebral foramina.		
5. Using a 72-in. SID, direct the central ray 15–20° cephalad through C-4.	The central ray should enter at or slightly inferior to the level of the most prominent point of the thyroid cartilage; the degree of angulation depends on the amount of cervical spine curvature.		
6. Center the cassette to the central ray.			
7. Collimate to the neck crosswise and to the film lengthwise; use gonadal shielding.			
8. Make the exposure during suspended respiration.			

CRITICAL ANATOMY: Intervertebral foramina and pedicles of the side furthest from the film.

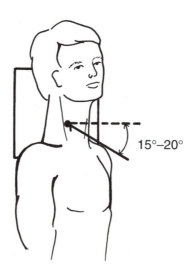

FIGURE 10–3. LPO cervical spine.

NOTES

▶ LATERAL CERVICAL SPINE

OBJECTIVE: After practice, each student will position a patient for a lateral projection of the cervical spine.

PATIENT PREP: Remove hairpins, dental appliances, earrings, necklaces, glasses, and bra; gown the patient.

FILM: 10 in. × 12 in. or 8 in. × 10 in. lengthwise, grid or non-grid.

TASK ANALYSIS		CORRECTLY PERFORMED?	
MAJOR STEPS	KEY INFORMATION	YES	NO
1. Assist the patient to the lateral erect position in front of the upright grid device.	The patient should look straight ahead while sitting or standing with the arms at the sides. The projection may also be obtained with the patient supine on the table, using a horizontal beam.		
2. Using a 72-in. SID, direct the central ray perpendicular and centered to the grid device.	A 72-in. SID minimizes magnification produced by the increased OID.		
3. Center the coronal plane passing through the EAM to the midline of the upright grid device.	The patient's adjacent shoulder should rest against the upright grid device for support.		
4. Rotate the patient's shoulders posteriorly (for patients with normal kyphosis).	If the patient is round-shouldered, the shoulders should be rotated anteriorly.		
5. Adjust the shoulders so a line drawn between them is perpendicular to the film plane.	The interpupillary line should also be perpendicular to the film.		
6. Adjust the body to a true lateral position.	The long axis of the cervical spine should be parallel to the film plane, with no leaning.		
7. Elevate the chin slightly.	The acanthiomeatal line should be parallel with the floor to prevent superimposition of the mandibular rami and the spine.		
8. Ask the patient to look steadily at one point on the wall to help maintain the position.			
9. Direct the central ray perpendicular to C-4.	The central ray should enter at the level of the superior border of the most prominent point of the thyroid cartilage.		
10. Center the cassette to the central ray.			

Continued

	TASK ANALYSIS	CORRECTLY PERFORMED?
MAJOR STEPS	KEY INFORMATION	YES NO

11. Depress the shoulders as much as possible and immobilize by suspending a sandbag from each wrist. | The sandbags should be of equal weight.

12. Collimate to the neck crosswise and to the film lengthwise; use gonadal shielding, if possible.

13. Make the exposure during suspended *expiration.* | Deep expiration helps obtain maximum depression of the shoulders.

CRITICAL ANATOMY: Vertebral bodies, intervertebral disk spaces, zygapophyseal joints of C-2 through C-7, articular pillars, and spinous processes.

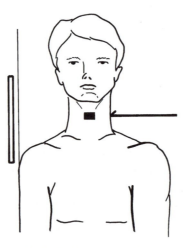

FIGURE 10–4. Lateral cervical spine.

NOTES

EVALUATOR SIGNATURE _____   DATE _____

► HYPERFLEXION–HYPEREXTENSION LATERAL CERVICAL SPINE

OBJECTIVE: After practice, each student will position a patient for hyperflexion and hyperextension lateral projections of the cervical spine.

PATIENT PREP: Remove hairpins, dental appliances, earrings, necklaces, glasses, and bra; gown the patient.

FILM: 10 in. × 12 in. or 8 in. × 10 in. lengthwise, grid or non-grid.

TASK ANALYSIS		CORRECTLY PERFORMED?	
MAJOR STEPS	KEY INFORMATION	YES	NO
1. Assist the patient to the erect lateral position in front of the upright grid device.	The patient should be positioned as for the neutral projection of the cervical spine and may be sitting or standing.		
2. Set the technical factors.			
3. a. *Hyperflexion:* Instruct the patient to drop the head forward, bringing the chin as close to the chest as possible.	Keep the midsagittal plane of the head parallel to the film plane for both projections.		
b. *Hyperextension:* Instruct the patient to elevate the chin as far as possible.	The patient should be looking up at the ceiling for the hyperextension projection.		
4. Using a 72-in. SID, direct the central ray perpendicular to C-4.	The central ray should enter at the level of the uppermost margin of the thyroid cartilage. A 72-in. SID is used to reduce magnification.		
5. Center the cassette to the central ray.			
6. Depress the shoulders and immobilize by suspending a sandbag from each wrist.	The sandbags should be of equal weight. Make sure the body is in a true lateral position.		
7. Collimate to the neck lengthwise and crosswise; use gonadal shielding, if possible.			
8. Make the exposure during suspended *expiration.*			

NOTE: *Normal anteroposterior movement or, as a result of disease or trauma, limited movement can be demonstrated through functional studies of this type. The spinous processes should be widely separated in the hyperflexion position and close together in the hyperextension position.*

CRITICAL ANATOMY: Zygapophyseal joints, cervical bodies, and intervertebral disk spaces.

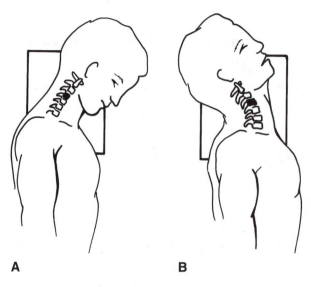

A   B

FIGURE 10–5. **A.** Hyperflexion. **B.** Hyperextension.

NOTES
....

EVALUATOR SIGNATURE _____ DATE _____

► LATERAL CERVICOTHORACIC SPINE (SWIMMER'S POSITION)

OBJECTIVE: After practice, each student will position a patient for a lateral projection of the cervicothoracic spine.

PATIENT PREP: Remove all clothing and jewelry above the waist; gown the patient.

FILM: 10 in. × 12 in. lengthwise, grid.

TASK ANALYSIS

MAJOR STEPS	KEY INFORMATION	CORRECTLY PERFORMED? YES NO
1. Assist the patient to the lateral recumbent position on the table.	This projection may also be obtained with the patient erect or supine with a horizontal beam.	
2. Center the midaxillary plane to the midline of the table.	Align the patient to the long axis of the table.	
3. Place supports under the head and lower thorax.	The long axis of the vertebral column should be parallel to the film plane.	
4. Raise the arm nearest the table above the head.	For this projection, the patient's cervicothoracic spine should remain in a nearly lateral position while one shoulder is moved anteriorly and the other is rotated posteriorly. This arm position prevents superimposition of the shoulders over this region.	
5. Position the arm furthest from the table at the patient's side, depressing the shoulder and rotating it slightly posteriorly.		
6. Readjust the body plane to the lateral position, if necessary.		
7. Direct the central ray 3–5° caudad to T-1.	The central ray should enter at the level of the suprasternal notch. Minimal angulation of the central ray is used to demonstrate the intervertebral disk spaces.	
8. Center the cassette to the central ray.		
9. Collimate to the spine crosswise and to the film size lengthwise; use gonadal shielding.		
10. Make the exposure during suspended respiration.		

CRITICAL ANATOMY: Vertebral bodies and intervertebral disk spaces from C-5 through T-4.

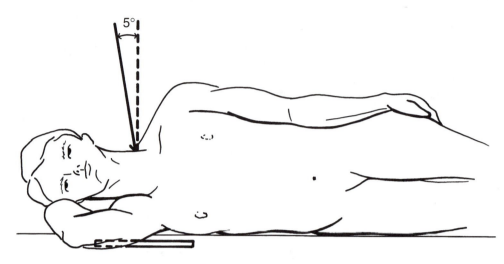

FIGURE 10–6. Lateral cervicothoracic spine.

NOTES
....

▶ AP THORACIC SPINE

OBJECTIVE: After practice, each student will position a patient for an AP projection of the thoracic spine.

PATIENT PREP: Remove all clothing and jewelry above the waist; gown the patient.

FILM: 14 in. × 17 in. or 7 in. × 17 in. lengthwise, grid.

TASK ANALYSIS		CORRECTLY PERFORMED?	
MAJOR STEPS	KEY INFORMATION	YES	NO
1. Position the patient supine with the body parallel to the long axis of the table.	To prevent accentuation of the thoracic curvature, the patient's head should rest directly on the table or on a thin pillow. The anode-heel effect can be used to produce a more uniform density; the patient's head should be placed near the anode.		
2. Center the midsagittal plane to the midline of the table.	Check body alignment from the head or foot of the table.		
3. Place the patient's arms along the sides of the body and check for rotation.	The shoulders should lie in the same transverse plane, parallel with the table.		
4. Flex the patient's knees and hips enough to place the lower back in contact with the table.	Sponges or pillows may be used to elevate and support the knees.		
5. Direct the central ray perpendicular to the level of T-7.	This point is approximately 3 to 4 in. inferior to the manubrial notch. The top of the cassette should be 1 1/2 to 2 in. above the top of the shoulders.		
6. Center the cassette to the central ray.			
7. Collimate to the spine crosswise and to the film size lengthwise; use gonadal shielding.			
8. Make the exposure during: a. Shallow breathing, or b. Suspended *expiration.*			

CRITICAL ANATOMY: Vertebral bodies, transverse processes, and intervertebral disk spaces.

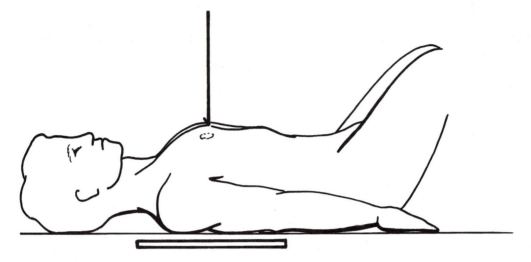

FIGURE 10–7. AP thoracic spine.

NOTES

▶ LATERAL THORACIC SPINE

OBJECTIVE: After practice, each student will position a patient for a lateral projection of the thoracic spine.

PATIENT PREP: Remove all clothing and jewelry above the waist; gown the patient.

FILM: 14 in. × 17 in. or 7 in. × 17 in. lengthwise, grid.

TASK ANALYSIS		CORRECTLY PERFORMED?	
MAJOR STEPS	KEY INFORMATION	YES	NO
1. Assist the patient to the left lateral recumbent position on the table.	The left lateral position will minimize the heart shadow; this projection may also be obtained with the patient erect.		
2. Place a firm pillow under the patient's head.	Raise the midsagittal plane of the head to the level of the long axis of the vertebral column.		
3. Center the midaxillary plane to the midline of the table.	Flex the knees to a comfortable position; the right knee should be directly over the left to help prevent rotation.		
4. Position the arms at right angles to the long axis of the body.	This arm placement elevates the ribs to provide a clear view of the intervertebral foramina and demonstrate the vertebrae distal to the glenohumeral joints.		
5. Adjust the body to a true lateral position.	Check for rotation from the head or foot of the table.		
6. Position a radiolucent support under the lower thoracic/waist region.	The long axis of the vertebral column should be parallel to the film plane.		
7. Direct the central ray perpendicular to the long axis of the spine at the level of T-7.	The level of T-7 is 5 to 6 in. inferior to the spinous process of C-7.		
8. Center the cassette to the central ray.			
9. Collimate to the thoracic spine crosswise and to the film size lengthwise; use gonadal shielding.			
10. Place lead masking on the table behind the patient.	The lead will absorb the scatter radiation coming from the patient and, therefore, improve radiographic contrast.		
11. Make the exposure during: a. Quiet breathing, or b. Suspended *expiration.*	Quiet breathing will help blur the lung and rib detail.		

CRITICAL ANATOMY: Spinous processes, vertebral bodies of T-3 through T-12, intervertebral foramina, pedicles, and intervertebral disk spaces.

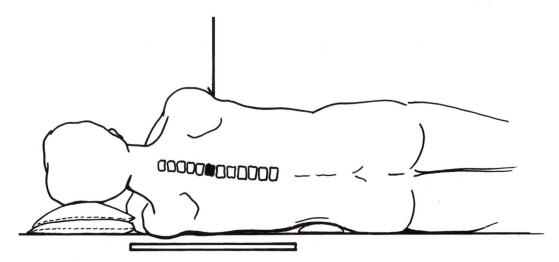

FIGURE 10–8. Lateral thoracic spine.

NOTES

EVALUATOR SIGNATURE _____ DATE _____

▶ AP LUMBAR SPINE

OBJECTIVE: After practice, each student will position a patient for an AP projection of the lumbar spine.

PATIENT PREP: Remove all clothing except shoes and socks; gown the patient.

FILM: 14 in. × 17 in. or 11 in. × 14 in. lengthwise, grid.

TASK ANALYSIS		CORRECTLY PERFORMED?	
MAJOR STEPS	KEY INFORMATION	YES	NO

MAJOR STEPS	KEY INFORMATION	YES	NO
1. Position the patient supine with the body parallel to the long axis of the table.			
2. Center the midsagittal plane to the midline of the table.	Check body alignment from the head or foot of the table.		
3. Check for rotation.	The shoulders should lie in the same transverse plane parallel to the table; small sponges may be needed to support one or both sides of the pelvis.		
4. Flex the patient's knees and hips.	Flexion places the back closer to the table, reducing the lordotic curve and improves delineation of the intervertebral disk spaces. The patient can lean the knees together for support. Sponges or pillows may be used to elevate and support the knees.		
5. Direct the central ray perpendicular to: a. L-4 (14 in. × 17 in. cassette).	L-4 is approximately 1/2 in. above the level of the iliac crests.		
b. L-3 (11 in. × 14 in. cassette).	L-3 is about 1/2 in. above the iliac crests.		
6. Center the cassette to the central ray.			
7. Collimate to the spine crosswise and to the film size lengthwise; use gonadal shielding, if possible.	Some department routines require collimation to the abdomen.		
8. Make the exposure during suspended *expiration.*			

CRITICAL ANATOMY: Vertebral bodies, transverse processes, lamina, and intervertebral disk spaces.

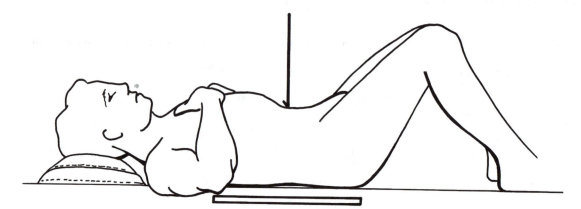

FIGURE 10–9. AP lumbar spine.

NOTES

EVALUATOR SIGNATURE _____ DATE _____

▶ AP OBLIQUE LUMBAR SPINE

OBJECTIVE: After practice, each student will position a patient for AP oblique projections of the lumbar spine.

PATIENT PREP: Remove all clothing except shoes and socks; gown the patient.

FILM: 10 in. × 12 in. or 11 in. × 14 in. lengthwise, grid.

TASK ANALYSIS		CORRECTLY PERFORMED?	
MAJOR STEPS	KEY INFORMATION	YES	NO
1. Assist the patient to the supine position on the table.			
2. Slide the patient approximately 4 in. toward one side of the table.	The patient should still be supine.		
3. Rotate the patient 45° toward the opposite side.	If the patient is moved to the left side of the table, he or she can be turned onto the right side and rolled backward to a 45° oblique position, using a lumbar sponge to support the shoulders and hips. The left arm should be brought across the chest with both hands kept near the head; the legs can also be used for support.		
4. Center the spine to the midline of the table.	The sagittal plane approximately 2 in. medial to the ASIS should be centered to the table.		
5. Direct the central ray perpendicular to the level of L-3.	L-3 is approximately 1 1/2 in. above the level of the iliac crests.		
6. Center the cassette to the central ray.			
7. Collimate to the spine crosswise and to the film size lengthwise; use gonadal shielding.			
8. Make the exposure during suspended *expiration*.			
9. Both oblique projections are obtained for comparison.			

CRITICAL ANATOMY: Zygapophyseal joints, pedicles, pars interarticularis, and superior and inferior articular processes nearest the film.

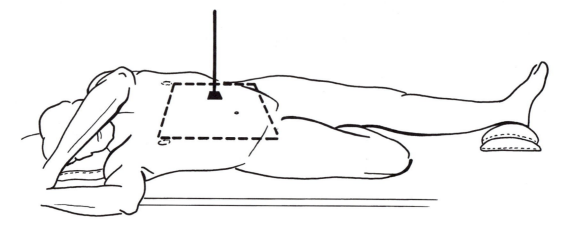

FIGURE 10–10. RPO lumbar spine.

NOTES

▶ LATERAL LUMBAR SPINE

OBJECTIVE: After practice, each student will position a patient for a lateral projection of the lumbar spine.

PATIENT PREP: Remove all clothing except shoes and socks; gown the patient using an open-back gown.

FILM: 14 in. × 17 in. or 11 in. × 14 in. lengthwise, grid.

TASK ANALYSIS		CORRECTLY PERFORMED?	
MAJOR STEPS	KEY INFORMATION	YES	NO
1. Assist the patient to the lateral recumbent position on the table.	The lateral projection obtained may depend on the department preference and the ability of the patient.		
2. Flex the patient's knees and hips just enough to achieve a comfortable position.			
3. Place a small sandbag or sponge between the knees.	The knees must be exactly superimposed; a sandbag or sponge will help prevent rotation.		
4. Center the midaxillary plane to the middle of the table.	Check body alignment from the head or foot of the table.		
5. Position a radiolucent support under the waist.	The long axis of the entire spine should be parallel with the film plane. Men with broad shoulders and narrow hips may need an additional support under the hips, whereas women with wide hips and narrow shoulders may need support under the shoulders. Palpate and look at the spinous processes to determine the need for supports.		
6. Adjust the patient's body to a true lateral position.	Check for rotation by looking down the patient's back. A plane passing through the shoulders, back, and pelvis should be perpendicular to the table.		
7. Direct the central ray perpendicular to: a. L-4 (14 in. × 17 in. cassette).	L-4 is about 1/2 in. above the level of the iliac crests.		
b. L-3 (11 in. × 14 in. cassette).	L-3 is about 1 1/2 in. above the iliac crests.		
8. Center the cassette to the central ray.			
9. Place lead shielding on the table behind the patient.	The lead will absorb excess scatter radiation coming from the patient and improve radiographic quality.		

Continued

TASK ANALYSIS		CORRECTLY PERFORMED?	
MAJOR STEPS	KEY INFORMATION	YES	NO

10. Collimate to the spine crosswise and to the film lengthwise.

11. Make the exposure during suspended *expiration.*

NOTE: *If a radiolucent support is not used under the waist, the central ray must be angled 5° caudad for males and 8° caudad for females.*

CRITICAL ANATOMY: Vertebral bodies, pedicles, intervertebral disk spaces, intervertebral foramina, and spinous processes.

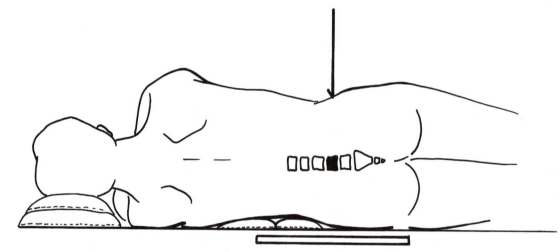

FIGURE 10–11. Lateral lumbar spine.

NOTES

EVALUATOR SIGNATURE _____ DATE _____

▶ AP AXIAL LUMBOSACRAL JUNCTION (L5–S1) & SACROILIAC JOINTS

OBJECTIVE: After practice, each student will position a patient for an AP axial projection of the lumbosacral junction and sacroiliac joints.

PATIENT PREP: Remove all clothing except shoes and socks; gown the patient.

FILM: 8 in. × 10 in. or 10 in. × 12 in. lengthwise, or 9 in. × 9 in., grid.

TASK ANALYSIS		CORRECTLY PERFORMED?	
MAJOR STEPS	KEY INFORMATION	YES	NO
1. Position the patient supine with the body parallel to the long axis of the table.			
2. Center the midsagittal plane to the midline of the table.	Check body alignment from the head or foot of the table.		
3. Check for rotation.	The shoulders should lie in the same transverse plane; small sponges may be needed to support one or both sides of the pelvis. *Do not* flex the knees and hips.		
4. Direct the central ray 30–35° cephalad to the level of the ASIS.	The amount of central ray angulation depends on the curvature of the lower back; usually 30° for males and 35° for females is appropriate.		
5. Center the cassette to the central ray.			
6. Collimate to a 5 in. × 5 in. field size; use gonadal shielding.			
7. Make the exposure during suspended *expiration.*			

NOTE: *When this projection is obtained to demonstrate the sacroiliac joints, the patient may be prone with the central ray directed caudad.*

CRITICAL ANATOMY: L5–S1 disk space and sacroiliac joints.

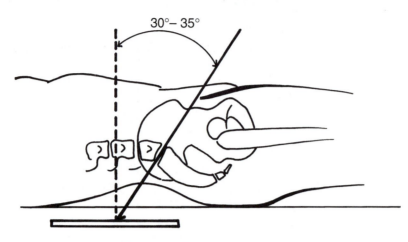

FIGURE 10–12. AP axial lumbosacral junction.

NOTES
....

EVALUATOR SIGNATURE _____ DATE _____

▶ LATERAL LUMBOSACRAL JUNCTION (L5–S1)

OBJECTIVE:	After practice, each student will position a patient for a lateral projection of the lumbosacral joint and sacroiliac joints.
PATIENT PREP:	Remove all clothing except shoes and socks; gown the patient using an open-back gown.
FILM:	8 in. × 10 in. lengthwise or 9 in. × 9 in., grid.

TASK ANALYSIS		CORRECTLY PERFORMED?	
MAJOR STEPS	KEY INFORMATION	YES	NO
1. Assist the patient to the lateral recumbent position on the table.	The lateral projection obtained may depend on the department preference and patient condition.		
2. Flex the patient's knees and hips just enough to achieve a comfortable position.			
3. Place a small sandbag or sponge between the knees.	The knees must be exactly superimposed; a sandbag or sponge will help prevent rotation.		
4. Center the coronal plane passing 1 1/2 in. posterior to the midaxillary plane to the middle of the table.	Check body alignment from the head or foot of the table.		
5. Position a radiolucent support under the waist.	The long axis of the entire spine should be parallel to the film plane. Men with broad shoulders and narrow hips may need an additional support under the hips, whereas women with wide hips and narrow shoulders may need support under the shoulders. Palpate and look at the spinous processes to determine the need for supports.		
6. Adjust the patient's body to a true lateral position.	Check for rotation by looking down the patient's back. A plane passing through the shoulders, back, and pelvis should be perpendicular to the table.		
7. Direct the central ray perpendicular to the the level of the transverse plane passing midway between the iliac crests and the ASIS.			
8. Center the cassette to the central ray.			

Continued

TASK ANALYSIS		CORRECTLY PERFORMED?	
MAJOR STEPS	**KEY INFORMATION**	**YES**	**NO**
9. Place lead shielding on the table behind the patient.	The lead will absorb excess scatter radiation coming from the patient and improve radiographic quality.		
10. Collimate to a 5 in. × 5 in. field size.			
11. Make the exposure during suspended *expiration.*			

NOTE: *If a radiolucent support is not used under the waist, the central ray is angled approximately 5° caudad for males and 8° caudad for females.*

CRITICAL ANATOMY: 5th vertebral body, L-5–S-1 intervertebral disk space, and 1st sacral segment.

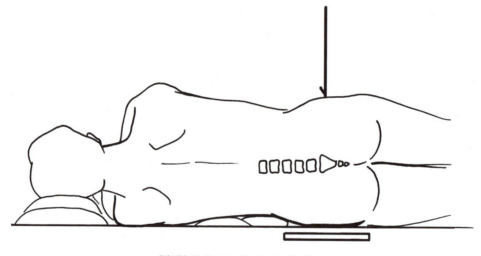

FIGURE 10–13. Lateral lumbosacral junction.

NOTES

EVALUATOR SIGNATURE _____ DATE _____

► AP SACRUM

OBJECTIVE: After practice, each student will position a patient for an AP projection of the sacrum.

PATIENT PREP: Remove all clothing except shoes and socks; gown the patient.

FILM: 10 in. × 12 in. lengthwise, grid.

TASK ANALYSIS		CORRECTLY PERFORMED?	
MAJOR STEPS	KEY INFORMATION	YES	NO

MAJOR STEPS	KEY INFORMATION
1. Position the patient supine with body parallel to the long axis of the table.	
2. Center the midsagittal plane to the midline of the table.	Check body alignment from the head or foot of the table.
3. Check for rotation.	The shoulders and hips should lie in the same transverse plane.
4. Adjust the pelvis to true anatomical position.	Small sponges may be needed to support one or both sides of the pelvis. A support may also be placed under the patient's knees to ease the stress on the back.
5. Direct the central ray 15° cephalad to the midpoint of the transverse plane passing midway between the symphysis pubis and the ASISs.	The central ray will enter approximately 2 in. superior to the symphysis pubis. The central ray angle may vary with the angulation of the sacral plane.
6. Center the cassette to the central ray.	
7. Collimate to include the ASISs crosswise and to the film lengthwise.	
8. Make the exposure during suspended *expiration.*	

CRITICAL ANATOMY: Sacral foramina and alae.

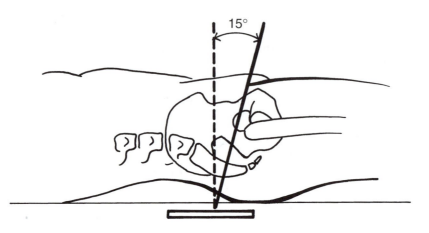

FIGURE 10–14. AP sacrum.

NOTES
....

▶ AP COCCYX

OBJECTIVE: After practice, each student will position a patient for an AP projection of the coccyx.

PATIENT PREP: Remove all clothing except shoes and socks; gown the patient.

FILM: 8 in. × 10 in. lengthwise or 9 in. × 9 in., grid.

TASK ANALYSIS		CORRECTLY PERFORMED?	
MAJOR STEPS	KEY INFORMATION	YES	NO

MAJOR STEPS	KEY INFORMATION
1. Position the patient supine with the body parallel to the long axis of the table.	
2. Center the midsagittal plane to the midline of the table.	Check body alignment from the head or foot of the table.
3. Check for rotation.	The shoulders and hips should lie in the same transverse plane.
4. Adjust the pelvis to true anatomical position.	Small sponges may be needed to support one or both sides of the pelvis. A support may also be placed under the patient's knees to ease the stress on the back.
5. Direct the central ray 10° caudad to a point 2 in. superior to the symphysis pubis.	The central ray angle may vary with the angulation of the coccygeal plane.
6. Center the cassette to the central ray.	
7. Collimate to a 4 in. × 5 in. field size.	
8. Make the exposure during suspended *expiration*.	

CRITICAL ANATOMY: Coccygeal segments.

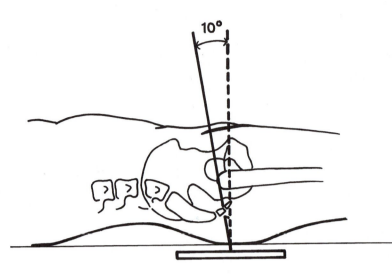

FIGURE 10–15. AP coccyx.

NOTES

▶ LATERAL SACRUM & COCCYX

OBJECTIVE: After practice, each student will position a patient for lateral projections of the sacrum and coccyx.

PATIENT PREP: Remove all clothing except shoes and socks; gown the patient using an open-back gown.

FILM: 10 in. × 12 in. (sacrum), 8 in. × 10 in. lengthwise or 9 in. × 9 in. (coccyx), grid.

TASK ANALYSIS		CORRECTLY PERFORMED?	
MAJOR STEPS	KEY INFORMATION	YES	NO

1. Assist the patient to the lateral recumbent position on the table.	The lateral projection obtained may depend on the department preference and the ability of the patient.		
2. Flex the patient's knees and hips just enough to achieve a comfortable position.			
3. Position a radiolucent support under the waist.	The long axis of the entire spine should be parallel to the film plane. Men with broad shoulders and narrow hips may need an additional support under the hips, whereas women with wide hips and narrow shoulders may need support under the shoulders. Feel and look at the spinous processes to determine the need for supports.		
4. Adjust the patient's body to a true lateral position.	Check body alignment from the head or foot of the table. The plane of the shoulders, back, and pelvis should be perpendicular to the table.		
5. Adjust the arms to form a right angle with the body.			

6. *Sacrum:*
    a. Center the coronal plane passing 3 in. posterior to the midaxillary plane to the table.
    b. Direct the central ray perpendicular to the level of the ASIS.			

7. *Coccyx:* a. Center the coronal plane 5 in. posterior to the midaxillary plane to the midline of the table.	The coccyx can be palpated at the base of the spine and should be centered to the midline of the table and cassette.		

Continued

TASK ANALYSIS		CORRECTLY PERFORMED?	
MAJOR STEPS	KEY INFORMATION	YES	NO

b. Direct the central ray perpendicular to the level of the coccyx.

8. Center the cassette to the central ray.

9. Collimate to an 8 in. × 10 in. field size (sacrum) or a 4 in. × 5 in. field size (coccyx).

10. Place lead shielding on the table behind the patient.   The lead will absorb excessive scatter radiation coming from the patient and improve film quality.

11. Make the exposure during suspended *expiration*.

CRITICAL ANATOMY: *Sacrum*—Sacral promontory, sacral canal, sacral spine, and sacral segments. *Coccyx*—Coccygeal segments and cornua.

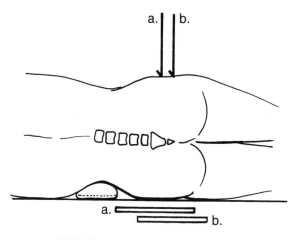

FIGURE 10–16. Lateral sacrum (a) and coccyx (b).

NOTES

EVALUATOR SIGNATURE _____ DATE _____

SKULL

11

▶ AP AXIAL (GRASHEY–TOWNE) SKULL

OBJECTIVE: After practice, each student will position a patient for an AP axial projection of the cranium using the Grashey–Towne method.

PATIENT PREP: Remove all opaque objects from the head and neck region, including jewelry, hairpins, hairpieces, and dental appliances.

FILM: 10 in. × 12 in. lengthwise, grid.

TASK ANALYSIS		CORRECTLY PERFORMED?	
MAJOR STEPS	KEY INFORMATION	YES	NO

1. Set technical factors.	The patient position may be difficult to maintain.		
2. Position the patient supine on the table or seated with the back to an upright grid device.	The upright position is more comfortable for the hypersthenic patient and facilitates patient positioning without increasing object–image receptor distance.		
3. Center the midsagittal plane to the midline of the table or the upright grid device.			
4. Adjust the shoulders to lie in the same plane.	Make sure the patient's body is parallel with the long axis of the table.		
5. Position the patient's arms comfortably at the sides.			
6. Adjust the patient's head so the midsagittal plane is perpendicular to the film plane.			
7. Tuck the chin down so the orbitomeatal line is perpendicular to the film plane; if this is not possible, adjust the head so the infraorbitomeatal line is perpendicular to the film plane.	Immobilize the head with head clamps and/or tape, if necessary.		
8. Center the cassette so the upper border is just above the top of the head.			
9. Direct the central ray through the foramen magnum: a. 30° caudad to the orbitomeatal line. b. 37° caudad to the infraorbitomeatal line.	The central ray passes through a line connecting both EAMs and should project the dorsum sellae through the foramen magnum.		

Continued

TASK ANALYSIS		CORRECTLY PERFORMED?	
MAJOR STEPS	KEY INFORMATION	YES	NO

10. Collimate to include the vertex and ears; use gonadal shielding.

11. Make the exposure during suspended respiration.

CRITICAL ANATOMY: Occipital bone, lambdoidal suture, foramen magnum, and dorsum sellae with posterior clinoid processes.

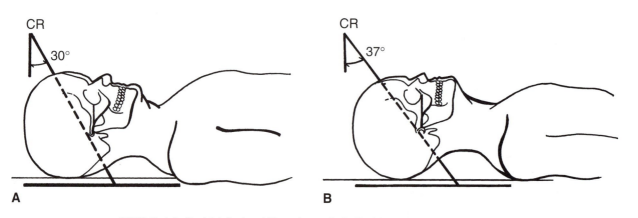

FIGURE 11–1. **A.** AP axial skull using a 30° central ray angle. **B.** AP axial skull using a 37° central ray angle.

NOTES

EVALUATOR SIGNATURE _____ DATE _____

▶ PA AXIAL (HAAS) SKULL

OBJECTIVE: After practice, each student will position a patient for a PA axial projection of the skull using the Haas method.

PATIENT PREP: Remove all opaque objects from the head and neck region, including jewelry, hairpins, hairpieces, and dental appliances.

FILM: 10 in. × 12 in. lengthwise, grid.

TASK ANALYSIS		CORRECTLY PERFORMED?	
MAJOR STEPS	KEY INFORMATION	YES	NO
1. Set the technical factors.	The patient position may be difficult to maintain.		
2. Position the patient prone on the table or seated facing an upright grid device.			
3. Center the midsagittal plane to the midline of the table or the upright grid device.			
4. Adjust the shoulders to lie in the same transverse plane, parallel with the film plane.	If the patient is prone, position the arms in a comfortable position with the elbows flexed.		
5. Position the patient's forehead and nose on the table or the upright grid device with the midsagittal plane perpendicular to the midline of the grid.			
6. Adjust the flexion of the head so the orbitomeatal line is perpendicular to the film plane.	In the prone position, a sponge or other support may be used to elevate the upper thorax of thin patients and make them more comfortable. Immobilize the head with head clamps, if necessary.		
7. Direct the central ray 25° cephalad to a point 1 1/2 in. above the nasion.	The central ray will enter approximately 1 1/2 in. below the inion.		
8. Center the cassette to the central ray.			
9. Collimate to include the vertex and ears; use gonadal shielding.			
10. Make the exposure during suspended respiration.			

NOTE: *This position is the reverse of the AP axial (Grashey/Towne) projection and should be used for hypersthenic or other patients who are unable to assume the AP position.*

CRITICAL ANATOMY: Occipital bone, dorsum sellae, foramen magnum, and lambdoidal suture.

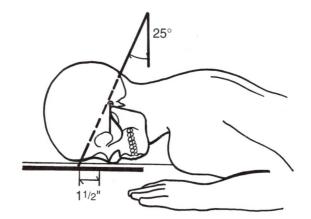

FIGURE 11–2. PA axial skull.

▶ PA SKULL

OBJECTIVE: After practice, each student will position a patient for a PA projection of the cranium.

PATIENT PREP: Remove all opaque objects from the head and neck region, including jewelry, hairpins, hairpieces, and dental appliances.

FILM: 10 in. × 12 in. lengthwise, grid.

TASK ANALYSIS		CORRECTLY PERFORMED?	
MAJOR STEPS	KEY INFORMATION	YES	NO
1. Set the technical factors.	The patient position may be difficult to maintain.		
2. Position the patient prone on the table or seated facing an upright grid device.			
3. Center the midsagittal plane to the midline of the table or the upright grid device.			
4. Adjust the shoulders to lie in the same transverse plane, parallel with the film plane.	If the patient is prone, place the arms in a comfortable position with the elbows flexed.		
5. Rest the patient's forehead and nose on the table or upright grid device with the midsagittal plane perpendicular to the film plane.			
6. Adjust the head so the orbitomeatal line is perpendicular to the film plane.	In the prone position, a sponge or other support may be used to elevate the upper thorax of thin patients and make them more comfortable. Immobilize the head with head clamps, if necessary.		
7. Direct the central ray:			
a. 15° caudad to exit at the nasion.	Preferred for a general survey examination of the skull; sometimes referred to as a PA Caldwell skull projection.		
b. Perpendicular to the nasion.	Performed when the frontal bone is the primary area of interest.		
c. 20–25° caudad through the midorbits.	Demonstrates the superior orbital fissures.		
d. 25–30° caudad to the nasion.	Demonstrates the rotundum foramina.		

Continued

TASK ANALYSIS		CORRECTLY PERFORMED?	
MAJOR STEPS	KEY INFORMATION	YES	NO

8. Center the cassette to the central ray.

9. Collimate to include the vertex and ears; use gonadal shielding.

10. Make the exposure during suspended respiration.

CRITICAL ANATOMY: Frontal bone and crista galli.

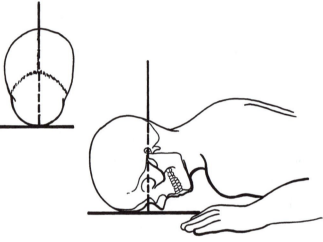

FIGURE 11–3. PA skull.

NOTES

▶ LATERAL SKULL

OBJECTIVE: After practice, each student will position a patient for a lateral projection of the skull.

PATIENT PREP: Remove all opaque objects from the head and neck region, including jewelry, hairpins, hairpieces, and dental appliances.

FILM: 10 in. × 12 in. crosswise, grid.

TASK ANALYSIS		CORRECTLY PERFORMED?	
MAJOR STEPS	KEY INFORMATION	YES	NO

1. Set the technical factors.	The patient position may be difficult to maintain.		
2. Position the patient semiprone on the table or seated facing an upright grid device.	Patients who have labored breathing or are unable to hold still in the recumbent position should be radiographed in the upright position.		
3. Position the patient's head with the side of interest against the table or upright grid device and the ear centered to the midline of the grid.	When on the table, the patient's right arm should be at the side and the left arm resting near the head (right lateral); the patient may support self with the left forearm and flexed leg.		
4. Adjust the rotation of the body so the midsagittal plane of the head is parallel to the film plane and the interpupillary line is perpendicular to the film plane.	On the table, head clamps or sponges may be needed to elevate and immobilize the head and/or mandible.		
5. Adjust the head flexion so the infraorbitomeatal line is parallel to the transverse axis of the film.			
6. Direct the central ray perpendicular to the cassette through the point: a. **Entire skull:** Midway between the inion and the glabella. b. **Sella turcica:** 3/4 in. anterior and superior to the external acoustic meatus.	Adjust head centering so structure of interest is centered to the midline of the grid device.		
7. Center the cassette to the central ray.	Make sure the top of the cassette is at least 1 in. above the top of the skull.		
8. Recheck the patient position to make sure the head is not rotated.			
9. Collimate to include the vertex, C-1, inion, and glabella; use gonadal shielding.			

Continued

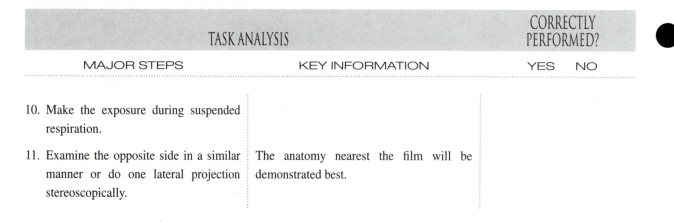

TASK ANALYSIS		CORRECTLY PERFORMED?	
MAJOR STEPS	KEY INFORMATION	YES	NO

10. Make the exposure during suspended respiration.			
11. Examine the opposite side in a similar manner or do one lateral projection stereoscopically.	The anatomy nearest the film will be demonstrated best.		

NOTE: *For patients who are unable to sit upright or lie in a semiprone position, cross-table lateral projections may be obtained with the patient lying supine on the table; this method is recommended for trauma patients. Positioning accuracy may be evaluated by checking to see if the temporomandibular joints are exactly superimposed; any separation indicates rotation or tilt in the direction of the separation.*

CRITICAL ANATOMY: Sella turcica and parietal bones.

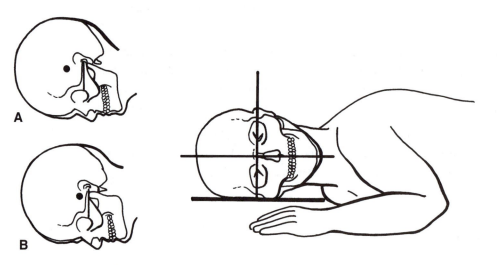

FIGURE 11–4. Lateral skull; centering for entire skull (**A**) and sella turcica (**B**).

NOTES

EVALUATOR SIGNATURE _____ DATE _____

► SUBMENTOVERTICAL (FULL BASAL) SKULL

OBJECTIVE: After practice, each student will position a patient for a submentovertical (full basal) projection of the skull.

PATIENT PREP: Remove all opaque objects from the head and neck region, including jewelry, hairpins, hairpieces, and dental appliances.

FILM: 10 in. × 12 in. lengthwise, grid.

TASK ANALYSIS		CORRECTLY PERFORMED?	
MAJOR STEPS	KEY INFORMATION	YES	NO
1. Set technical factors.	The patient position may be difficult to maintain.		
2. Assist the patient to the AP seated, erect position in front of an upright grid device; center the body and head to the midline of the grid.	Although the patient will be more comfortable in the erect position, this examination may be performed with the patient supine, the body adequately elevated on pillows, and the knees flexed to permit complete extension of the head.		
3. Lean the head backward and rest the vertex against the midline of the upright grid device so that, as nearly as possible, the infraorbitomeatal line is parallel to the film plane.	Using the hand, support the patient's back and/or head as the patient leans backward.		
4. Adjust the head so the midsagittal plane is perpendicular to the film plane.			
5. Direct the central ray perpendicular to the infraorbitomeatal line through a point midway between the angles of the mandible.	The central ray may need to be angled slightly cephalad so it is perpendicular to the infraorbitomeatal line.		
6. Center the cassette to the central ray.			
7. Collimate to include the nose, ears, and posterior skull; use gonadal shielding.			
8. Make the exposure during suspended respiration.			

NOTE: *When the exposure factors are decreased, this projection can be used to demonstrate the zygomatic arches; the central ray is directed perpendicular to the infraorbitomeatal line between the zygomatic arches through the coronal plane passing 1 in. posterior to the outer canthi.*

CRITICAL ANATOMY: Foramen magnum, petrous portions, mandible, and sphenoid sinuses.

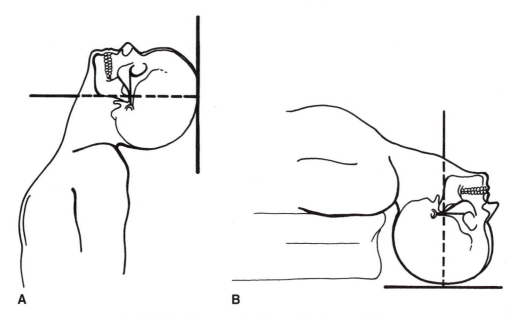

FIGURE 11–5. Submentovertical skull, erect **(A)** and recumbent **(B)**.

NOTES

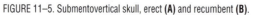

EVALUATOR SIGNATURE _____ DATE _____

► VERTICOSUBMENTAL (FULL BASAL) SKULL

OBJECTIVE: After practice, each student will position a patient for a verticosubmental (full basal) projection of the skull.

PATIENT PREP: Remove all opaque objects from the head and neck region, including jewelry, hairpins, hairpieces, and dental appliances.

FILM: 10 in. × 12 in. lengthwise, grid.

TASK ANALYSIS		CORRECTLY PERFORMED?	
MAJOR STEPS	KEY INFORMATION	YES	NO
1. Set technical factors.	The patient position may be difficult to maintain.		
2. Position the patient prone on the table.			
3. Center the midsagittal plane of the head and body to the midline of the table.			
4. Adjust the shoulders to lie in the same plane, parallel with the film plane.	Place the patient's arms in a comfortable position with the elbows flexed.		
5. Hyperextend the neck and head; rest the patient's head on the chin.			
6. Adjust the head so the midsagittal plane is perpendicular to the film plane.	Use head clamps to immobilize the head.		
7. Direct the central ray perpendicular to the infraorbitomeatal line through the sella turcica.	The central ray should pass through a point 3/4 in. anterior to the external acoustic meatus.		
8. Center the cassette to the central ray.			
9. Collimate to include the nose, ears, and posterior skull; use gonadal shielding.			
10. Make the exposure during suspended respiration.			

NOTE: *This projection provides an elongated, reverse view of the basal skull projection and is performed when obtaining the submentovertical projection is contraindicated by the patient's condition.*

CRITICAL ANATOMY: Foramen magnum, petrous portions, mandible, and sphenoid sinuses.

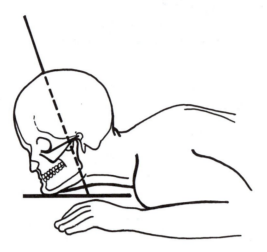

FIGURE 11–6. Verticosubmental skull.

NOTES
....

▶ MODIFIED LATERAL (LAW) SKULL FOR PETROUS PORTIONS

OBJECTIVE: After practice, each student will position a patient for a modified lateral projection of the skull to demonstrate the petrous portions using the Law method.

PATIENT PREP: Remove all opaque objects from the head and neck region, including jewelry, hairpins, hairpieces, and dental appliances.

FILM: 8 in. × 10 in. crosswise or 9 in. × 9 in., grid.

TASK ANALYSIS		CORRECTLY PERFORMED?	
MAJOR STEPS	KEY INFORMATION	YES	NO
1. Set the technical factors.	The patient position may be difficult to maintain.		
2. Position the patient semiprone on the table or seated facing an upright grid device.	Place the arms in a comfortable position.		
3. Adjust the head so the interpupillary line is perpendicular to the film plane, the infraorbitomeatal line is parallel with the transverse axis of the film and the midsagittal plane is parallel with the film plane.	The head should be in a true lateral position.		
4. Position the head so the midsagittal plane is rotated 15° toward the cassette from a true lateral position.	The patient's head will be in a "natural" position.		
5. Center the point 1 in. directly posterior to the external acoustic meatus of the side down to the midline of the table or upright grid device.	The auricle may be folded forward and held in place by the weight of the patient's head or with tape.		
6. Direct the central ray 15° caudad to the midpoint of the dependent mastoid.	The central ray will enter approximately 1 in. posterior and 2 in. superior to the opposite (side up) external acoustic meatus.		
7. Center the cassette to the central ray.			
8. Collimate to a 5 in. × 6 in. field size; use gonadal shielding.			
9. Make the exposure during suspended respiration.			
10. Examine the opposite side in a similar manner.	Both sides are obtained for comparison.		

NOTE: *A 15° angle board can be used to eliminate the central ray angle.*

CRITICAL ANATOMY: Mastoid air cells, internal and external acoustic meatuses, and lateral pars petrosa.

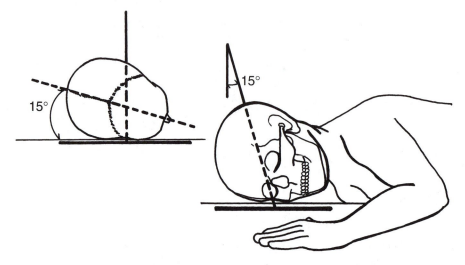

FIGURE 11–7. Modified lateral petrous portions.

NOTES
....

▶ AXIOLATERAL OBLIQUE (MAYER) SKULL FOR PETROUS PORTIONS

OBJECTIVE: After practice, each student will position a patient for an axiolateral oblique projection of the skull to demonstrate the petrous portions using the Mayer method.

PATIENT PREP: Remove all opaque objects from the head and neck region, including jewelry, hairpins, hairpieces, and dental appliances.

FILM: 8 in. × 10 in. lengthwise or 9 in. × 9 in., grid.

TASK ANALYSIS		CORRECTLY PERFORMED?	
MAJOR STEPS	KEY INFORMATION	YES	NO
1. Set the technical factors.	The patient position may be difficult to maintain.		
2. Position the patient supine on the table or seated with the back to an upright grid device.			
3. Rotate the head toward the side being examined, placing the midsagittal plane at a 45° angle to the film plane.	The ear of the side being examined should be closest to the film and that petrous ridge should be perpendicular to the film plane.		
4. Center the point directly behind the external acoustic meatus at the junction of the auricle and head of the side nearest the film to the midline of the table or upright grid device.	The auricle may be taped forward to remove the shadow from the mastoid area.		
5. Adjust the flexion of the head and neck to place the infraorbitomeatal line parallel to the transverse axis of the film.			
6. Direct the central ray 45° caudad through the dependent external acoustic meatus.			
7. Center the cassette to the central ray.			
8. Collimate to a 5 in. × 8 in. field size; use gonadal shielding.			
9. Make the exposure during suspended respiration.			
10. Examine the opposite side in a similar manner.	Both sides are obtained for comparison.		

NOTE: *There are numerous modifications of this projection that involve increased rotation of the head toward the lateral position and a smaller central ray angle. Department procedure manuals should be consulted for consistency.*

CRITICAL ANATOMY: Mastoid air cells, EAM, bony labyrinth, and mastoid antrum.

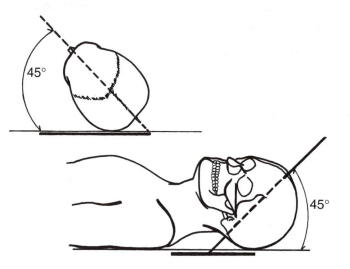

FIGURE 11–8. Axiolateral oblique petrous portions.

NOTES
....

▶ POSTERIOR PROFILE (STENVERS) SKULL FOR PETROUS PORTIONS

OBJECTIVE: After practice, each student will position a patient for a posterior profile projection of the skull to demonstrate the petrous portions using the Stenvers method.

PATIENT PREP: Remove all opaque objects from the head and neck region, including jewelry, hairpins, hairpieces, and dental appliances.

FILM: 8 in. × 10 in. crosswise or 9 in. × 9 in., grid.

TASK ANALYSIS		CORRECTLY PERFORMED?	
MAJOR STEPS	KEY INFORMATION	YES	NO
1. Set the technical factors.	The patient position may be difficult to maintain.		
2. Position the patient prone on the table or seated facing an upright grid device.	Place the arms in a comfortable position.		
3. Position the patient's forehead, nose, and cheek ("three-point landing") on the table or the upright grid device.	The side nearest the film will be examined.		
4. Adjust the head flexion so the infraorbitomeatal line is parallel with the transverse axis of the film.			
5. Adjust the head rotation so the midsagittal plane and the film plane form a 45° angle.	Use head clamps or sponges and sandbags to immobilize, if necessary.		
6. Center the point 1 in. directly anterior to the external acoustic meatus to the midline of the grid device.			
7. Direct the central ray 12° cephalad to the level of the external acoustic meatus.			
8. Center the cassette to the central ray.			
9. Collimate to a 5 in. × 7 in. field size; use gonadal shielding.			
9. Make the exposure during suspended respiration.			
10. Examine the opposite side in a similar manner.	Both sides are obtained for comparison.		

NOTE: *For patients unable to sit or lie prone, the reverse projection (Arcelin) may be performed with a 10° caudad central ray angle directed to the side furthest from the film.*

CRITICAL ANATOMY: Profile projection of the petrous pyramid nearest the film, mastoid air cells, petrous ridge, mastoid process, and internal acoustic canal.

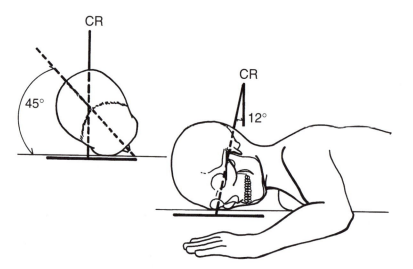

FIGURE 11–9. Posterior profile petrous portions.

NOTES
....

▶ ANTERIOR PROFILE (ARCELIN) SKULL FOR PETROUS PORTIONS

OBJECTIVE: After practice, each student will position a patient for an anterior profile projection of the skull to demonstrate the petrous portions using the Arcelin method.

PATIENT PREP: Remove all opaque objects from the head and neck region, including jewelry, hairpins, hairpieces, and dental appliances.

FILM: 8 in. × 10 in. crosswise or 9 in. × 9 in., grid.

TASK ANALYSIS		CORRECTLY PERFORMED?	
MAJOR STEPS	KEY INFORMATION	YES	NO
1. Set the technical factors.	The patient position may be difficult to maintain.		
2. Position the patient supine on the table.	Place the arms in a comfortable position.		
3. Center the midsagittal plane of the patient's body to the midline of the table.	The patient's body should be parallel with the long axis of the table.		
4. Check for rotation by making sure the shoulders lie in a plane parallel to the film.			
5. Rotate the head away from the side being examined so the midsagittal and film planes form a 45° angle.	The side of interest is furthest from the film.		
6. Center the point 1 in. directly anterior to the external acoustic meatus to the midline of the grid device.			
7. Adjust the head flexion so the infraorbitomeatal line is parallel with the transverse axis of the film.	Use head clamps, tape, or sponges and sandbags to immobilize, if necessary.		
8. Direct the central ray 10° caudad through the level of the external acoustic meatus.	The central ray should enter the cheek approximately 3/4 in. superior to the infraorbitomeatal line.		
9. Center the cassette to the central ray.			
10. Collimate to a 5 in. × 7 in. field size; use gonadal shielding.			
11. Make the exposure during suspended respiration.			
12. Examine the opposite side in a similar manner.	Both sides are obtained for comparison.		

NOTE: *This projection is a reverse of the Stenvers method and produces a similar result. It is used for adults and children who cannot be positioned prone or seated erect. Note, however, that the eye dose is greater in the anterior versus the posterior projection.*

CRITICAL ANATOMY: Profile projection of the petrous pyramid furthest from the film, mastoid air cells, petrous ridge, mastoid process, and internal acoustic canal.

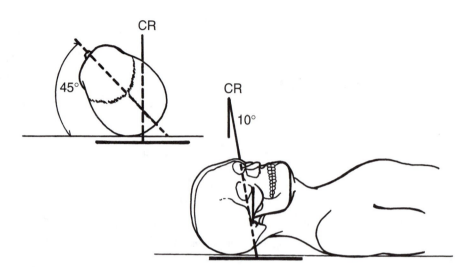

FIGURE 11–10. Anterior profile petrous portions.

NOTES
....

EVALUATOR SIGNATURE _____ DATE _____

FACIAL BONES & PARANASAL SINUSES

► PA (CALDWELL) PARANASAL SINUSES

OBJECTIVE: After practice, each student will position a patient for a PA projection of the paranasal sinuses using the Caldwell method.

PATIENT PREP: Remove all opaque objects from the head and neck region, including jewelry, hairpins, hairpieces, and dental appliances.

FILM: 8 in. × 10 in. lengthwise or 9 in. × 9 in., grid or non-grid.

TASK ANALYSIS		CORRECTLY PERFORMED?	
MAJOR STEPS	KEY INFORMATION	YES	NO

MAJOR STEPS	KEY INFORMATION	YES	NO
1. Seat the patient facing an upright grid device.			
2. Center the midsagittal plane to the midline of the upright grid device.			
3. Position the shoulders so they lie in the same transverse plane, parallel with the film.	The patient's arms should be in a comfortable position.		
4. Position the patient's forehead and nose against the upright grid device with the midsagittal plane perpendicular to the film plane.			
5. Adjust the head flexion so the orbitomeatal line is perpendicular to the film plane.			
6. Direct the central ray 15° caudad, exiting at the nasion.	The original Caldwell method used a 23° caudad angle to the glabellomeatal line. Because this position is difficult to maintain, the position was modified. *Note:* This projection may also be obtained by angling the cassette 15° and directing the central ray horizontally, better demonstrating any existing air–fluid levels.		
7. Center the cassette to the central ray.			
8. Collimate to a 6 in. × 6 in. field size; use gonadal shielding.			
9. Make the exposure during suspended respiration.			

CRITICAL ANATOMY: Frontal sinuses and anterior ethmoid sinuses.

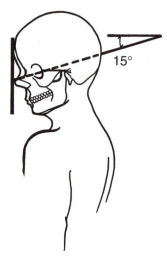

FIGURE 12–1. PA paranasal sinuses.

NOTES
....

▶ PARIETOACANTHIAL (WATERS) PARANASAL SINUSES

OBJECTIVE: After practice, each student will position a patient for a parietoacanthial projection of the paranasal sinuses using the Waters method.

PATIENT PREP: Remove all opaque objects from the head and neck region, including jewelry, hairpins, hairpieces, and dental appliances.

FILM: 8 in. × 10 in. lengthwise or 9 in. × 9 in., grid or non-grid.

TASK ANALYSIS		CORRECTLY PERFORMED?	
MAJOR STEPS	KEY INFORMATION	YES	NO
1. Set the technical factors.	The patient position may be difficult to maintain.		
2. Seat the patient facing an upright grid device.	The patient's arms should be positioned comfortably at the sides; this projection must be done upright to demonstrate air–fluid levels.		
3. Center the midsagittal plane to the midline of the upright grid device.			
4. Position the patient's shoulders so they lie in the same transverse plane, parallel with the film plane.	The arms should be in a comfortable position.		
5. Place the patient's head on the extended chin with the midsagittal plane perpendicular to the midline of the grid device.			
6. Adjust the head flexion so the orbitomeatal line and the film plane form a 37° angle.	Use a protractor or other device as a guide. On an average person, the mentomeatal line will be perpendicular to the film plane and the tip of the nose should be approximately 1/2 in. from the table. Use head clamps to immobilize, if necessary.		
7. Direct the central ray horizontally, exiting at the acanthion.			
8. Center the cassette to the central ray.			
9. Collimate to a 6 in. × 6 in. field size; use gonadal shielding.			
10. Make the exposure during suspended respiration.	For department routines that require it, the patient's mouth is opened prior to the exposure for demonstration of the sphenoid sinuses.		

NOTE: *When the head is correctly positioned, the petrous ridges will be projected just below the maxillary sinuses.*

CRITICAL ANATOMY: Maxillary sinuses and sphenoid sinuses (if the mouth is open).

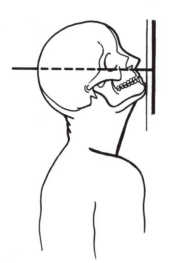

FIGURE 12–2. Parietoacanthial paranasal sinuses.

NOTES

▶ LATERAL PARANASAL SINUSES

OBJECTIVE: After practice, each student will position a patient for a lateral projection of the paranasal sinuses.

PATIENT PREP: Remove all opaque objects from the head and neck region, including jewelry, hairpins, hairpieces, and dental appliances.

FILM: 8 in. × 10 in. lengthwise or 9 in. × 9 in., grid or non-grid.

TASK ANALYSIS		CORRECTLY PERFORMED?	
MAJOR STEPS	KEY INFORMATION	YES	NO
1. Set the technical factors.	The patient position may be difficult to maintain.		
2. Seat the patient obliquely facing an upright grid device.			
3. Position the patient's head so the affected side is against the upright grid device.	The patient's arms should be in a comfortable position.		
4. Place the head in a true lateral position with the midsagittal plane parallel to and the interpupillary line perpendicular with the film plane.			
5. Adjust the head flexion so the infraorbitomeatal line is parallel with the transverse axis of the film.			
6. Direct the central ray horizontally to a point 1/2 in. posterior to the outer canthus of the eye.			
7. Center the cassette to the central ray.	The cassette should be centered to the level of the canthi.		
8. Collimate to include the temporomandibular joint, nose, maxilla, and forehead; use gonadal shielding.			
9. Make the exposure during suspended respiration.			

NOTE: *This projection is similar to the lateral skull projection with the exception of the central ray location and technical factors. If this projection is used for preoperative measurement, precise positioning is critical and a 72-in. SID must be used to minimize magnification.*

CRITICAL ANATOMY: Frontal, ethmoid, sphenoid, and maxillary sinuses.

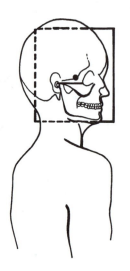

FIGURE 12–3. Lateral paranasal sinuses.

NOTES

EVALUATOR SIGNATURE _____ DATE _____

► SUBMENTOVERTICAL PARANASAL SINUSES (SMV)

OBJECTIVE: After practice, each student will position a patient for a submentovertical projection of the paranasal sinuses.

PATIENT PREP: Remove all opaque objects from the head and neck region, including jewelry, hairpins, hairpieces, and dental appliances.

FILM: 8 in. × 10 in. crosswise or 9 in. × 9 in., grid.

TASK ANALYSIS		CORRECTLY PERFORMED?	
MAJOR STEPS	KEY INFORMATION	YES	NO
1. Set the technical factors.	The patient position may be difficult to maintain.		
2. Assist the patient to the AP seated, erect position in front of an upright grid device with the body and head centered to the midline of the grid.			
3. Adjust the shoulders so they are in the same plane, parallel with the film plane.	Place the arms in a comfortable position.		
4. Extend the patient's head and neck and rest the vertex against the upright grid device.			
5. Adjust the head flexion so the infraorbitomeatal line is parallel with the film plane.			
6. Position the head so the midsagittal plane is perpendicular to the film plane and centered to the midline of the grid.	Use head clamps or tape to immobilize, if necessary.		
7. Direct the central ray perpendicular to the infraorbitomeatal line through the coronal plane passing 1 in. anterior to the external acoustic meatuses.	Angulation of the central ray may be necessary if the patient cannot adequately extend the head.		
8. Center the cassette to the central ray.			
9. Collimate to include the nose and external acoustic meatuses; use gonadal shielding.	Field size should be approximately 5 in. × 6 in.		
10. Make the exposure during suspended respiration.			

NOTE: *This projection is the same as the submentovertical basal skull projection with the exception of the central ray location.*

CRITICAL ANATOMY: Sphenoid and posterior ethmoid sinuses.

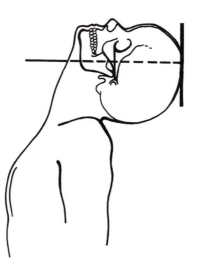

FIGURE 12–4. Submentovertical paranasal sinuses.

NOTES
....

EVALUATOR SIGNATURE _____ DATE _____

▶ PA FACIAL BONES

OBJECTIVE: After practice, each student will position a patient for a PA projection of the facial bones.

PATIENT PREP: Remove all opaque objects from the head and neck region, including jewelry, hairpins, hairpieces, and dental appliances.

FILM: 8 in. × 10 in. lengthwise or 9 in. × 9 in., grid.

TASK ANALYSIS		CORRECTLY PERFORMED?	
MAJOR STEPS	KEY INFORMATION	YES	NO
1. Set the technical factors.	The position may be difficult to maintain.		
2. Position the patient prone on the table or seated facing an upright grid device.			
3. Center the midsagittal plane to the midline of the table or upright grid device.			
4. Position the shoulders so they lie in the same transverse plane, parallel with the film plane.	If the patient is prone, flex the elbows and place the arms in a comfortable position with the hands near the shoulders.		
5. Position the patient's forehead and nose on the table or upright grid device with the midsagittal plane perpendicular to the film plane.			
6. Adjust the head so the orbitomeatal line is perpendicular to the film plane.			
7. Direct the central ray to exit at the acanthion, angling according to the area of interest:			
a. *General survey:* 15° caudad.	Projects the petrous ridges into the lower one third of the orbits.		
b. *Orbits:* 25° caudad.	Projects the petrous ridges clear of the orbits; centering may be to the level of the orbits, per department routine.		
c. *Mandibular rami:* Perpendicular.	Projects the petrous ridges into the entire orbit.		
8. Center the cassette to the central ray.			
9. Collimate to a 6 in. × 8 in. field size; use gonadal shielding.	The orbits and entire mandible should be included in the collimated field.		
10. Make the exposure during suspended respiration.			

CRITICAL ANATOMY: *15° angle*—Upper two thirds of the orbits and lower two thirds of the mandibular rami. *25° angle*—Orbital margins. *Perpendicular*—Maxillae, mandibular rami, and lateral portions of mandible.

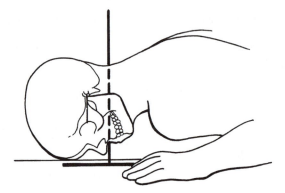

FIGURE 12–5. PA facial bones, 0° central ray angle.

NOTES

EVALUATOR SIGNATURE _____   DATE _____

▶ PARIETOACANTHIAL (WATERS) FACIAL BONES

OBJECTIVE: After practice, each student will position a patient for a parietoacanthial projection of the facial bones using the Waters method.

PATIENT PREP: Remove all opaque objects from the head and neck region, including jewelry, hairpins, hairpieces, and dental appliances.

FILM: 8 in. × 10 in. lengthwise or 9 in. × 9 in., grid.

TASK ANALYSIS		CORRECTLY PERFORMED?	
MAJOR STEPS	KEY INFORMATION	YES	NO
1. Position the patient prone on the table or seated facing an upright grid device.			
2. Center the midsagittal plane to the midline of the table or upright grid device.			
3. Adjust the shoulders so they lie in the same plane, parallel with the film.	If the patient is prone, flex the elbows and place the arms in a comfortable position with the hands near the shoulders.		
4. Place the patient's head on the extended chin rest with the midsagittal plane perpendicular to the midline of the grid device.			
5. Extend the head and neck so the orbitomeatal line forms a 37° angle with the film plane.	A protractor or other device can be used as a guide. On the average adult, the mentomeatal line will be perpendicular to the film plane and the tip of the nose will be approximately 1/2 in. from the table. Use head clamps to immobilize, if necessary.		
6. Direct the central ray perpendicular to the film, exiting at the acanthion.			
7. Center the cassette to the central ray.			
8. Collimate to include the orbits and mandible; use gonadal shielding.			
8. Make the exposure during suspended respiration.			

NOTE: *This exact projection is also obtained routinely in the upright position as part of a sinus examination. By decreasing the extension of the head slightly, this projection can be modified to better demonstrate a blow-out fracture.*

CRITICAL ANATOMY: Orbits, bony nasal septum, zygomatic arches, maxillae, and coronoid processes of the mandible.

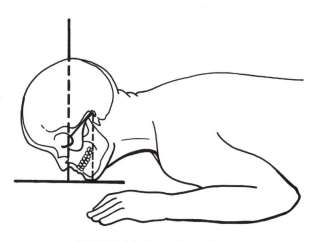

FIGURE 12–6. Parietoacanthial facial bones.

NOTES

EVALUATOR SIGNATURE _____ DATE _____

► LATERAL FACIAL BONES

OBJECTIVE: After practice, each student will position a patient for a lateral projection of the facial bones.

PATIENT PREP: Remove all opaque objects from the head and neck region, including jewelry, hairpins, hairpieces, and dental appliances.

FILM: 8 in. × 10 in. lengthwise or 9 in. × 9 in., grid.

TASK ANALYSIS		CORRECTLY PERFORMED?	
MAJOR STEPS	KEY INFORMATION	YES	NO
1. Set the technical factors.	The patient position may be difficult to maintain.		
2. Position the patient semiprone on the table or seated facing an upright grid device.	The patient will be in the RAO or LAO position.		
3. Position the patient's head so the affected side is nearest the table or upright grid device.	The patient's arms should be in a comfortable position.		
4. Adjust the rotation of the body so the midsagittal plane of the head is parallel to the film plane and the interpupillary line is perpendicular to the film plane.	If the patient is prone, the arm and leg can be flexed and used for support.		
5. Position the head so the infraorbitomeatal line is parallel with the transverse axis of the film.	Sponges may be needed to elevate and immobilize the head and/or mandible of the recumbent patient.		
6. Center the zygoma to the midline of the grid device.			
7. Direct the central ray perpendicular to the film through the zygoma.			
8. Center the cassette to the central ray.			
9. Collimate to include the temporomandibular joints, nose, mandible, and orbits; use gonadal shielding.			
10. Make the exposure during suspended respiration.			

NOTE: *This projection is similar to the lateral skull projection with the exception of the central ray location and technical factors.*

CRITICAL ANATOMY: Superimposed mandibular rami, mandible, coronoid processes, condylar processes, alveolar processes, and mandibular notches; maxillae, orbits, and nasal bones.

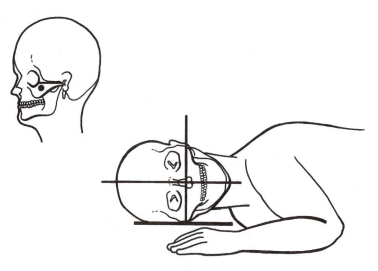

FIGURE 12–7. Lateral facial bones.

NOTES
....

▶ PARIETO-ORBITAL OBLIQUE (RHESE) OPTIC CANAL/FORAMEN

OBJECTIVE: After practice, each student will position a patient for a parieto-orbital oblique projection of the optic foramen using the Rhese method.

PATIENT PREP: Remove all opaque objects from the head and neck region, including jewelry, hairpins, hairpieces, and dental appliances.

FILM: 8 in. × 10 in. crosswise or 9 in. × 9 in., grid.

TASK ANALYSIS		CORRECTLY PERFORMED?	
MAJOR STEPS	KEY INFORMATION	YES	NO
1. Set the technical factors.	The patient position may be difficult to maintain.		
2. Position the patient semiprone on the table or seated facing an upright grid device.			
3. Adjust the shoulders so they lie in the same plane, parallel with the film.	If the patient is prone, flex the elbows and place the arms in a comfortable position with the hands near the shoulders.		
4. Position the patient's cheek, nose, and chin on the table or upright grid device.			
5. Center the orbit to the midline of the grid device.	The side of interest is nearest the film.		
6. Flex the head and neck so the acanthiomeatal line is parallel with the transverse axis of the film.			
7. Rotate the head so the midsagittal plane and the film plane form a 53° angle.	Use a protractor or other angle indicator to ensure accurate positioning. Use head clamps, tape, sponges, or sandbags to immobilize. *Precise positioning is important.*		
8. Direct the central ray perpendicular to the level of the outer canthus nearest the film.			
9. Center the cassette to the central ray.			
10. Collimate to include both orbits; use gonadal shielding.			
11. Make the exposure during suspended respiration.			
12. Examine the opposite side in a similar manner.	Both sides are obtained for comparison.		

NOTE: *The optic foramen should be seen in the lower outer quadrant of the orbit. Any lateral or longitudinal shifting of the foramen indicates incorrect rotation or head flexion.*

CRITICAL ANATOMY: Optic foramen of dependent side and orbital margins.

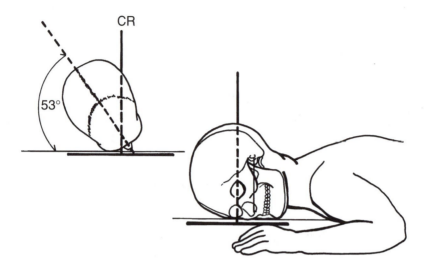

FIGURE 12–8. Parieto-orbital oblique optic foramen.

NOTES
....

▶ LATERAL NASAL BONES

OBJECTIVE: After practice, each student will position a patient for lateral projections of the nasal bones.

PATIENT PREP: Remove all opaque objects from the head and neck region, including jewelry, hairpins, hairpieces, and dental appliances.

FILM: 8 in. × 10 in. or 9 in. × 9 in. masked crosswise, non-grid.

TASK ANALYSIS		CORRECTLY PERFORMED?	
MAJOR STEPS	KEY INFORMATION	YES	NO
1. Set the technical factors.	The patient position may be difficult to maintain.		
2. Position the patient semiprone on the table.	The patient's head may rest on the right or left side, as both lateral projections are obtained.		
3. Rotate the body and head so the midsagittal plane of the head is parallel to the film plane.	The patient's arms should be in a comfortable position to help support the body.		
4. Adjust the head so the interpupillary line is perpendicular to the film plane.			
5. Position the head so the infraorbitomeatal line is parallel with the transverse axis of the film.	Sponges may be needed to elevate and immobilize the head and/or mandible of the recumbent patient.		
6. Center the nasion to the unmasked half of the cassette.	The projections should be on the film so they are facing away from each other.		
7. Secure the appropriate lead marker on the cassette anterior to the glabella, within the collimated field.			
8. Direct the central ray perpendicular to the cassette through a point 3/4 in. distal to the nasion.			
9. Collimate to include the nasion, acanthion, and soft-tissue structures of the nose; use gonadal shielding.	Make sure the lead marker is included in the collimation field.		
10. Make the exposure during suspended respiration.			
11. Examine the opposite side in a similar manner.			

NOTE: *Technical factors should allow visualization of both the soft tissue and bony structures; a soft-tissue technique might be used on one projection with a slightly darker technique on the other.*

CRITICAL ANATOMY: Nasal bones, anterior nasal spine of the maxilla, and the frontonasal junction.

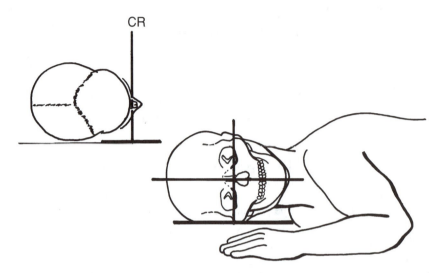

FIGURE 12–9. Lateral nasal bones.

NOTES
....

► SUBMENTOVERTICAL ZYGOMATIC ARCHES (SMV)

OBJECTIVE: After practice, each student will position a patient for a submentovertical projection of the zygomatic arches.

PATIENT PREP: Remove all opaque objects from the head and neck region, including jewelry, hairpins, hairpieces,
and dental appliances.

FILM: 8 in. × 10 in. crosswise or 9 in. × 9 in., non-grid or grid.

TASK ANALYSIS		CORRECTLY PERFORMED?	
MAJOR STEPS	KEY INFORMATION	YES	NO
1. Set the technical factors.	The patient position may be difficult to maintain.		
2. Assist the patient to the AP seated, erect position in front of an upright grid device with the body and head centered to the midline of the grid.	Although the patient is generally more comfortable in the erect position, this examination may be performed with the patient supine, the body adequately elevated on pillows, and the knees flexed to permit complete extension of the head.		
3. Adjust the shoulders so they are in the same plane, parallel with the film plane.	Place the arms in a comfortable position.		
4. Hyperextend the patient's head and neck and rest the vertex against the upright grid device.			
5. Adjust the head position so the infraorbitomeatal line is parallel with the film plane.			
6. Adjust the head so the midsagittal plane is perpendicular to the film plane and centered to the midline of the grid.	Use head clamps or tape to immobilize, if necessary.		
7. Direct the central ray perpendicular to the infraorbitomeatal line to a point midway between the gonia at the level of the zygomatic arches.	The central ray should pass through the coronal plane approximately 1 in. posterior to the outer canthi. A cephalic central ray angle is required if the patient cannot attain the desired postion.		
8. Center the cassette to the central ray.			
9. Collimate to include both zygomatic arches; use gonadal shielding.	Field size should be approximately 8 in. × 4 in.		
10. Make the exposure during suspended respiration.			

NOTE: *This projection is the same as the submentovertical basal skull projection with the exception of the central ray location. A decrease in exposure factors must be used.*

CRITICAL ANATOMY: Zygomatic arches, bilaterally.

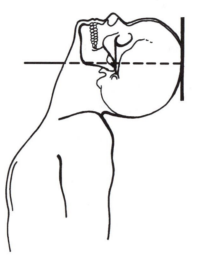

FIGURE 12–10. Submentovertical zygomatic arches.

NOTES
....

EVALUATOR SIGNATURE _____   DATE _____

► TANGENTIAL ZYGOMATIC ARCHES

OBJECTIVE: After practice, each student will position a patient for tangential projections of the zygomatic arches.

PATIENT PREP: Remove all opaque objects from the head and neck region, including jewelry, hairpins, hairpieces, and dental appliances.

FILM: 8 in. × 10 in. crosswise or 9 in. × 9 in. masked in half, non-grid or grid.

TASK ANALYSIS		CORRECTLY PERFORMED?	
MAJOR STEPS	KEY INFORMATION	YES	NO
1. Set the technical factors.	The patient position may be difficult to maintain.		
2. Assist the patient to the AP seated, erect position in front of an upright grid device with the body and head centered to the midline of the grid.	Although the patient is generally more comfortable in the erect position, this examination may be performed with the patient supine, the body adequately elevated on pillows, and the knees flexed to permit complete extension of the head.		
3. Adjust the shoulders so they are in the same plane, parallel with the film plane.	The arms should be in a comfortable position.		
4. Extend the patient's head and neck and rest the vertex against the upright grid device.			
5. Adjust the head position so the infraorbitomeatal line is parallel with the film plane.			
6. Rotate the patient's head toward the side of interest so the midsagittal plane is rotated 15°.	The side being examined will be closest to the film. Use head clamps or tape to immobilize, if necessary.		
7. Center the zygomatic arch to the unmasked half of the cassette (or to the grid device).			
8. Direct the central ray to the zygomatic arch at a right angle to the infraorbitomeatal line.	If, due to patient condition, the infraorbitomeatal line is not parallel to the film plane, angle the central ray accordingly.		
9. Center the cassette to the central ray.			
10. Collimate to the zygomatic arch nearest the film; use gonadal shielding.			

Continued

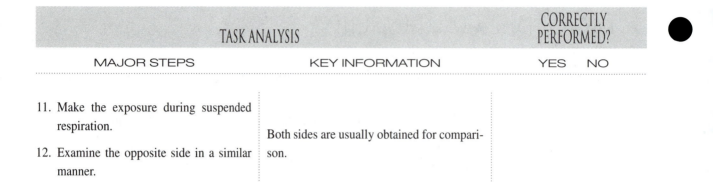

TASK ANALYSIS		CORRECTLY PERFORMED?	
MAJOR STEPS	KEY INFORMATION	YES	NO

11. Make the exposure during suspended respiration.	Both sides are usually obtained for comparison.		
12. Examine the opposite side in a similar manner.			

NOTE: *Depressed fractures or "flat" cheekbones usually are best demonstrated with this projection.*

CRITICAL ANATOMY: Zygomatic arch, unilateral.

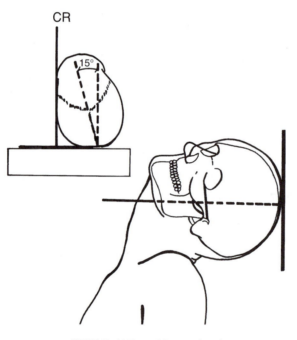

FIGURE 12–11. Tangential zygomatic arch.

NOTES
....

EVALUATOR SIGNATURE _____ DATE _____

► SUPEROINFERIOR (MODIFIED TITTERINGTON) ZYGOMATIC ARCHES

OBJECTIVE: After practice, each student will position a patient for a superoinferior projection of the zygomatic arches using the modified Titterington method.

PATIENT PREP: Remove all opaque objects from the head and neck region, including jewelry, hairpins, hairpieces, and dental appliances.

FILM: 8 in. × 10 in. lengthwise or 9 in. × 9 in., grid.

TASK ANALYSIS		CORRECTLY PERFORMED?	
MAJOR STEPS	KEY INFORMATION	YES	NO
1. Set the technical factors.	The patient position may be difficult to maintain.		
2. Position the patient prone on the table or seated facing a upright grid device.			
3. Center the midsagittal plane to the midline of the table or upright grid device.			
4. Adjust the shoulders so they are in the same plane, parallel with the film plane.	The arms should be in a comfortable position; if the patient is prone, the hands should be near the shoulders.		
5. Position the patient's chin on the midline of the table or upright grid device and adjust the neck extension so the nose is just barely touching the table.			
6. Position the head so the midsagittal plane is perpendicular to the film plane.	Immobilize with head clamps, if necessary.		
7. Direct the central ray 23–38° caudad to the mental point of the chin.	The central ray should pass between the zygomatic arches.		
8. Center the cassette to the central ray.			
9. Collimate to include the orbits and mandible; use gonadal shielding.			
10. Make the exposure during suspended respiration.			

NOTE: *The projection is similar to the parietoacanthial (Waters) projection except for the central ray angle and precise head flexion.*

CRITICAL ANATOMY: Zygomatic arches, bilaterally.

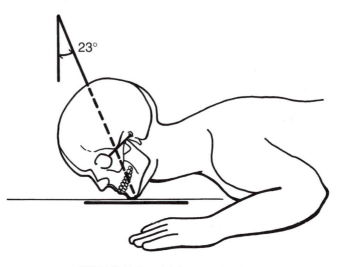

FIGURE 12–12. Superoinferior zygomatic arches.

NOTES

▶ PA AXIAL MANDIBULAR CONDYLES

OBJECTIVE: After practice, each student will position a patient for a PA axial projection of the mandible.

PATIENT PREP: Remove all opaque objects from the head and neck region, including jewelry, hairpins, hairpieces, and dental appliances.

FILM: 8 in. × 10 in. lengthwise or 9 in. × 9 in., grid.

TASK ANALYSIS		CORRECTLY PERFORMED?	
MAJOR STEPS	KEY INFORMATION	YES	NO
1. Set the technical factors.	The patient position may be difficult to maintain.		
2. Position the patient prone on the table or seated facing an upright grid device.			
3. Center the midsagittal plane to the midline of the table or upright grid device.			
4. Adjust the shoulders so they lie in the same plane, parallel with the film.	If the patient is prone, flex the elbows and place the arms in a comfortable position with the hands near the shoulders.		
5. Position the patient's forehead and nose on the table or upright grid device so the midsagittal plane is perpendicular to the film plane.	Use head clamps to immobilize the head, if necessary.		
6. Center the cassette to the level of the glabella.			
7. Direct the central ray 25–30° cephalad to the midpoint of the cassette.	The central ray should pass through a point just superior to the nasion.		
8. Collimate to a 6 in. × 8 in. field size; use gonadal shielding.			
9. Make the exposure during suspended respiration.			

NOTE: *This projection is basically the same as the PA axial (Haas) skull projection. The PA facial bone projection with a 0° angle can also be used to demonstrate any medial or lateral displacement of fractures of the mandibular rami.*

CRITICAL ANATOMY: Mandibular condyles and rami.

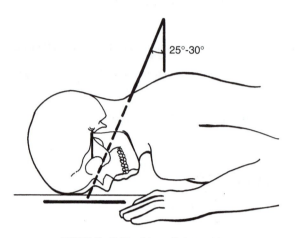
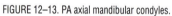

FIGURE 12–13. PA axial mandibular condyles.

NOTES

► AXIOLATERAL OBLIQUE MANDIBLE

OBJECTIVE: After practice, each student will position a patient for axiolateral oblique projections of the mandible.

PATIENT PREP: Remove all opaque objects from the head and neck region, including jewelry, hairpins, hairpieces, and dental appliances.

FILM: 8 in. × 10 in. lengthwise or 9 in. × 9 in., non-grid.

TASK ANALYSIS		CORRECTLY PERFORMED?	
MAJOR STEPS	KEY INFORMATION	YES	NO

1. Set the technical factors.	The patient position may be difficult to maintain.		
2. Position the patient semisupine on the table or seated obliquely facing an upright cassette holder.	If the patient is semisupine, support the body with sponges or pillows.		
3. Adjust the rotation of the body so the head can be placed in a lateral position on a cranially inclined cassette.	The patient's arms should be placed comfortably at the sides.		
4. Place the cassette crosswise on an angle sponge or board and position under the patient's cheek with the elevated side adjacent to the patient's shoulder.			
5. Center the side being examined to the cassette.	On the table, a sandbag should be placed at the superior end of the cassette for immobilization.		
6. Adjust the position of the head so the part of the mandible of greatest interest is parallel to the film plane: a. *Body:*			
1. Rotate the head so the body of the mandible is parallel with the film plane.	The patient's head should be rotated approximately 30° toward the cassette.		
2. Direct the central ray cephalad so the total angle (sponge/board and central ray) is approximately 25° and enters about 2 in. inferior to the gonion of the side up; adjust cassette centering, as necessary.	If no sponge or angle board is used, the central ray should be directed 25° cephalad.		

Continued

TASK ANALYSIS		CORRECTLY PERFORMED?	
MAJOR STEPS	KEY INFORMATION	YES	NO

b. ***Ramus:***

   1. Adjust the rotation of the head so the ramus of the side down is parallel to the film plane.

   2. Direct the central ray cephalad so the total angle (sponge/board and central ray) is approximately 30° and enters about 2 in. inferior to the gonion of the side up; adjust cassette centering, as necessary.

7. Collimate to include the entire mandible; use gonadal shielding.

8. Make the exposure during suspended respiration.

9. Examine the opposite side in a similar manner.

Key information:

The head should be nearly lateral relative to the film plane.

If no sponge or angle board is used, the central ray should be directed 30° cephalad.

Both sides are obtained for a complete study of the mandible.

NOTE: *If body or head rotation is contraindicated due to patient condition, the patient should be supine with the cassette supported in the vertical position adjacent to the mandible at the level of the occlusal plane. The central ray is then directed cross-table with a 30–35° cephalad and 10° anterior angle.*

CRITICAL ANATOMY: Condyle, mandibular notch, coronoid process, gonion, ramus, mandible, and alveolar process of the mandible (structures seen can vary with patient position).

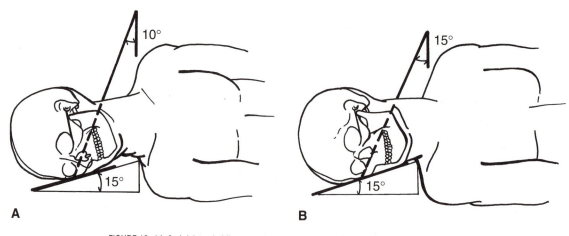

FIGURE 12–14. **A.** Axiolateral oblique mandibular body. **B.** Axiolateral oblique mandibular ramus.

EVALUATOR SIGNATURE _____ DATE _____

► AP AXIAL EXTRAORAL MANDIBULAR SYMPHYSIS

OBJECTIVE: After practice, each student will position a patient for an AP axial extraoral projection of the mandibular symphysis.

PATIENT PREP: Remove all opaque objects from the head, including jewelry, eyeglasses, and dental appliances.

FILM: 8 in. × 10 in. crosswise, 9 in. × 9 in. or occlusal film, non-grid.

TASK ANALYSIS		CORRECTLY PERFORMED?	
MAJOR STEPS	KEY INFORMATION	YES	NO
1. Assist the patient to a chair at the end of the table.	If the patient is unable to sit, the examination may be completed with the patient supine.		
2. Elevate the cassette or occlusal film on sponges, sandbags, or other support.	The film holder must be elevated to the approximate level of the patient's chin.		
3. Instruct the patient to rest the chin on the film holder.	The inferior surface of the chin should be in close contact with the film holder and positioned off-center distally to allow for the central ray angle.		
4. Adjust the head so the midsagittal plane is perpendicular to the film plane.			
5. Direct the central ray 40–45° toward the patient through the mandibular symphysis.	The central ray should enter between the lips and the tip of the chin.		
6. Align the film holder to the central ray.			
7. Collimate to the mandibular symphysis; use thyroid and gonadal shielding.	Make sure a right or left marker is on the film holder and within the collimated field.		
8. Make the exposure during suspended respiration.			

CRITICAL ANATOMY: Mandibular symphysis.

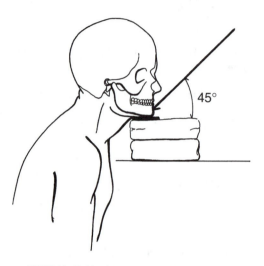

FIGURE 12–15. AP axial extraoral mandibular symphysis.

NOTES

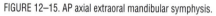

▶ AXIOLATERAL (SHULLER) TEMPOROMANDIBULAR JOINTS

OBJECTIVE: After practice, each student will position a patient for axiolateral projections of the temporo-mandibular joints using the Shuller method.

PATIENT PREP: Remove all opaque objects from the head and neck region, including jewelry, hairpins, hairpieces, and dental appliances.

FILM: 8 in. × 10 in. lengthwise or masked in half crosswise, 9 in. × 9 in., grid.

TASK ANALYSIS		CORRECTLY PERFORMED?	
MAJOR STEPS	KEY INFORMATION	YES	NO
1. Set the technical factors.	The patient position may be difficult to maintain.		
2. Position the patient semiprone on the table or seated obliquely facing an upright grid device.	Begin with the patient in the RAO position.		
3. Position the patient's head with the right side against the table or upright grid device.	Both sides must be examined with both the open and closed mouth (four exposures). The arms should be in a comfortable position.		
4. Center a point 1/2 in. anterior to the EAM to the midline of the grid.			
5. Adjust the head to place the midsagittal plane parallel to and the interpupillary line perpendicular to the film plane.	The head should be in a true lateral position with the infraorbitomeatal line parallel with the transverse axis of the film. Use head clamps or sponges to immobilize, if necessary.		
6. Direct the central ray 25–30° caudad through the dependent temporomandibular joint (side down).	The central ray will enter about 2–3 in. superior to the opposite temporomandibular joint.		
7. Center the cassette to the central ray.			
8. Collimate to the dependent temporomandibular joint; use gonadal shielding.	The collimation field should be no larger than 5 in. × 5 in.		
9. Make two separate exposures during suspended respiration: a. Mouth closed, and b. Mouth wide open.	A bite block may be used to immobilize the open mouth.		
10. Examine the opposite side in a similar manner.			

CRITICAL ANATOMY: Temporomandibular joint nearest the film; mandibular condyle and neck of the condylar process and temporomandibular fossa.

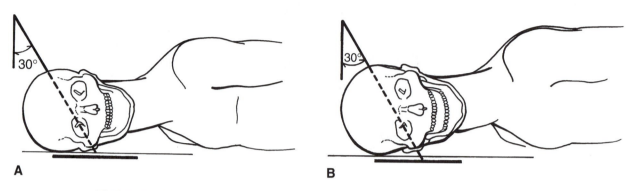

FIGURE 12–16**A**. Axiolateral temporomandibular joint, closed mouth. **B**. Axiolateral temporomandibular joint, open mouth.

NOTES

► AXIOLATERAL OBLIQUE TEMPOROMANDIBULAR JOINTS

OBJECTIVE: After practice, each student will position a patient for axiolateral oblique projections of the temporomandibular joints.

PATIENT PREP: Remove all opaque objects from the head and neck region, including jewelry, hairpins, hairpieces, and dental appliances.

FILM: 8 in. × 10 in. crosswise or 9 in. × 9 in., grid or non-grid.

TASK ANALYSIS		CORRECTLY PERFORMED?	
MAJOR STEPS	KEY INFORMATION	YES	NO
1. Set the technical factors.	The patient position may be difficult to maintain.		
2. Position the patient semiprone on the table or seated facing an upright grid device.	Begin with the patient in the RAO position.		
3. Position the patient's head with the right side against the table or upright grid device.	Both sides must be examined with both the open and closed mouth (four exposures). The arms should be in a comfortable position.		
4. Center a point 1/2 in. anterior to the EAM to the midline of the grid.			
5. From a true lateral position, rotate the head 15° toward the table so the head is resting comfortably on the cheek.	The head should be positioned similar to a Law projection, except the acanthiomeatal line should be parallel with the transverse axis of the film. Use head clamps to immobilize, if necessary.		
6. Direct the central ray 15° caudad through the dependent temporomandibular joint (side down).			
7. Center the cassette to the central ray.			
8. Collimate to the dependent temporomandibular joint; use gonadal shielding.	The collimation field should be no larger than 5 in. × 5 in.		
9. Make two separate exposures during suspended respiration: a. Mouth closed, and b. Mouth wide open.	A bite block may be used to immobilize the open mouth.		
10. Examine the opposite side in a similar manner.			

CRITICAL ANATOMY: Temporomandibular joint nearest the film; mandibular condyle and neck of the condylar process and temporomandibular fossa.

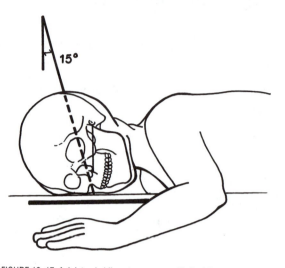

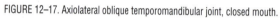

FIGURE 12–17. Axiolateral oblique temporomandibular joint, closed mouth.

NOTES
....

EVALUATOR SIGNATURE _____ DATE _____

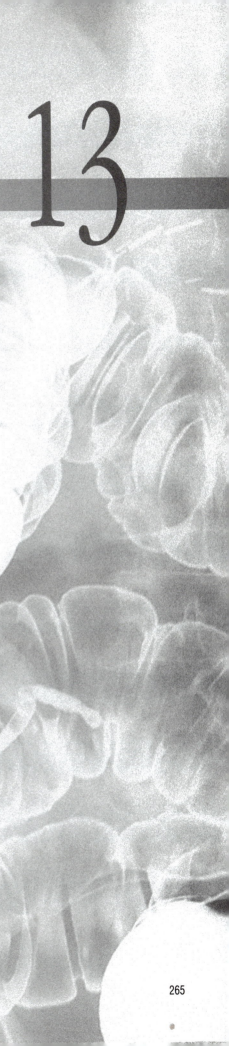

INTRODUCTION TO CONTRAST STUDIES

Radiography of the urinary, digestive, and biliary systems requires the administration of contrast media. The abdomen is an area of low subject contrast, given the similarity of the atomic numbers of the various abdominal structures. Positive contrast media, such as barium sulfate or water soluble iodine, have higher atomic numbers than the soft-tissue structures of the abdomen. Therefore, x-rays are more likely to be attenuated or absorbed within the contrast media, allowing for differentiation of contrast-filled structures. Negative contrast media, such as air, have lower atomic numbers than abdominal tissue and are frequently combined with positive contrast media for a double-contrast study. Double-contrast examinations are commonly performed on the stomach and large intestine.

▶ PATIENT PREPARATION

For most contrast studies, patient preparation begins before the day of the actual examination and may include fasting, a special diet, and/or laxatives or suppositories. For oral cholecystography, the patient must ingest the contrast medium the evening before the examination.

Acquisition of a relevant patient history is important for all radiographic examinations. For contrast studies, however, the history should include questions about the examination preparation (to ascertain whether it was followed correctly) and the allergy history (iodinated contrast media, only). Information obtained as part of the patient history should be communicated to the radiologist before the start of the procedure; this information may help with diagnosis or may result in modification of the procedure. For example, if vomiting or excessive diarrhea occurs following ingestion of the contrast medium for an oral cholecystogram, the contrast medium may be eliminated before it can be absorbed. When this occurs, the examination must be rescheduled or the patient may be scheduled for an ultrasound study of the gallbladder.

▶ ROOM PREPARATION

Radiographic examinations that require the use of contrast media generally require more accessory equipment than noncontrast media procedures. Although the list of necessary supplies varies depending on the procedure to be performed, it generally includes an emergency box or crash cart, disposable gloves, appropriate contrast medium, and administration equipment such as needles, syringes, cups, straws, or enema bag and tip. Because radiography of the digestive system generally includes fluoroscopy, the radiographer must be sure appropriate protective apparel, such as lead aprons, gloves, and thyroid shields, is available.

Because exposure to blood and body fluids is probable, cleanliness and the use of appropriate disinfectants to clean the radiographic table and ancillary equipment between patients are vitally important for preventing infection and disease transmission. Disposable gloves and a protective gown (if necessary) should be worn when contact with blood or body fluids is possible.

▶ RADIOGRAPHIC PROCEDURES

Radiographic examinations that require contrast media may be named according the structure being examined, physiologic function or region, or procedure for administration of contrast (Table 13–1). One or more of these terms will be used when describing the projections in the following chapters. Because body habitus determines the location of the abdominal organs of the digestive system, the radiographer should observe the television monitor during fluoroscopy to determine exact location of these structures; guidelines are included, however, in the following projections.

TABLE 13–1. Terms Used to Describe Equivalent Contrast Studies*

Structures Demonstrated	Function or Region	Administration
Kidneys, ureters, bladder	Excretory urogram (Ex.U.)	Intravenous pyelogram (IVP) or retrograde pyelogram
Esophagus	Barium swallow Esophagram	
Stomach (or stomach and esophagus)	Upper GI	
Small intestine	Small bowel follow-through (SBFT)	
Large intestine, colon	Large bowel	Barium enema (BE)
Gallbladder		Oral cholecystogram

*Although other examinations are performed of these anatomical areas, this table identifies most of the more common procedures.

URINARY SYSTEM

14

▶ AP PRE- & POST-CONTRAST URINARY TRACT (UROGRAM)

OBJECTIVE: After practice, each student will position a patient for an AP projection of the abdomen for a pre- or post-injection radiograph of the urinary tract.

PATIENT PREP: Remove all clothing except shoes and socks and gown the patient; determine if pre-examination instructions were followed and obtain a pertinent patient history.

FILM: 14 in. × 17 in. lengthwise, grid.

TASK ANALYSIS		CORRECTLY PERFORMED?	
MAJOR STEPS	KEY INFORMATION	YES	NO
1. Position the patient supine with the body parallel to the long axis of the table.	The shoulders and pelvis should be adjusted so there is no rotation; sponges may be used for support, if necessary.		
2. Center the midsagittal plane to the midline of the table.	Check body alignment from the head or foot of the table.		
3. Position the patient's arms comfortably at the sides.	Make sure the patient's arms are *not* resting on the abdomen or tucked under the body.		
4. Flex the knees and support them with sandbags, sponges, or pillows.	This eases the stress on the patient's back and makes the position more comfortable.		
5. Direct the central ray perpendicular to the level of the iliac crests.			
6. Center the cassette to the central ray.	The bladder and symphysis pubis should be included on this film. If the patient is tall, a separate radiograph of the kidney area should be included.		
7. Collimate to the abdominal walls laterally and to the film size lengthwise; use gonadal shielding, if possible.			
8. Make the exposure during suspended *expiration.*			

NOTE: *Ureteral compression may be used for post-injection films to enhance the visualization of the renal pelves and calyces. Prone or upright films may also be performed.*

CRITICAL ANATOMY: *Pre-injection radiograph*—Renal shadows, inferior margin of the liver, and psoas major muscles. *Post-injection radiograph*— Highlighted renal cortex and medullary tissue, opacified renal calyces, renal pelves, ureters, and bladder.

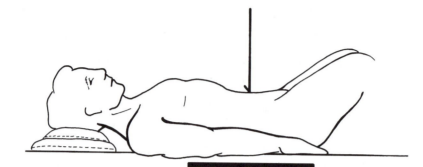

FIGURE 14–1. AP urogram.

NOTES
....

EVALUATOR SIGNATURE _____   DATE _____

▶ AP COLLIMATED RENAL AREA (UROGRAM)

OBJECTIVE: After practice, each student will position a patient for a collimated AP projection of the renal area for a pre- or post-contrast radiograph of the urinary tract.

PATIENT PREP: Remove all clothing except shoes and socks and gown the patient; determine if pre-examination instructions were followed and obtain a pertinent patient history.

FILM: 11 in. × 14 in. or 10 in. × 12 in. crosswise, grid.

TASK ANALYSIS

MAJOR STEPS	KEY INFORMATION	CORRECTLY PERFORMED? YES	NO
1. Position the patient supine with the body parallel to the long axis of the table.	The shoulders and pelvis should be adjusted so there is no rotation; sponges may be used for support, if necessary.		
2. Center the midsagittal plane to the midline of the table.	Check body alignment from the head or foot of the table.		
3. Position the patient's arms comfortably at the sides.	Make sure the patient's arms are *not* resting on the abdomen or tucked under the body.		
4. Flex the knees and support them with sandbags, sponges, or pillows.	This eases the stress on the patient's back and makes the position more comfortable.		
5. Direct the central ray perpendicular to the transverse plane halfway between the xiphoid process and the iliac crests.	Approximately 1 in. of the iliac crests will be seen on the finished radiograph.		
6. Center the cassette to the central ray.	Both kidneys must be completely included on the film; check the preliminary film to determine kidney location.		
7. Collimate to the abdominal walls laterally and to include the iliac crests lengthwise; use gonadal shielding.	The top of the gonadal shield should be at the level of the ASIS.		
8. Make the exposure during suspended *expiration*.			

NOTE: *Ureteral compression may be used for post-injection films to enhance the visualization of the renal pelves and calyces.*

CRITICAL ANATOMY: *Preliminary film*—Renal shadows, psoas major muscles, and transverse processes of the spine. *Post-injection film*—Highlighted renal cortex and medullary tissue, major and minor calyces, renal pelves, and proximal ureters (varies depending on the post-injection time and renal function).

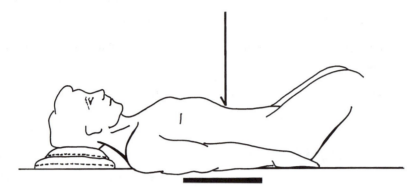

FIGURE 14–2. AP collimated renal area.

NOTES
....

▶ AP OBLIQUE URINARY TRACT (UROGRAM)

OBJECTIVE: After practice, each student will position a patient for AP oblique projections of the abdomen as performed for an urogram.

PATIENT PREP: Remove all clothing except shoes and socks and gown the patient; determine if pre-examination instructions were followed and obtain a pertinent patient history.

FILM: 14 in. × 17 in. lengthwise, grid.

TASK ANALYSIS		CORRECTLY PERFORMED?	
MAJOR STEPS	KEY INFORMATION	YES	NO
1. Assist the patient to the supine position on the table.			
2. Slide the patient toward one side of the table approximately 3 in.	The patient should still be supine.		
3. Rotate the patient 30° toward the opposite side.	If the patient is moved to the left side of the table, he or she can turn onto the right side and roll backward to a 30° oblique position, using a lumbar sponge to support the shoulders and hips. The left arm should be brought across the chest with both hands kept near the head; the legs can also be used for support.		
4. Center the sagittal plane approximately 3 in. medial to the elevated ASIS to the midline of the table.	Align the patient to the long axis of the table.		
5. Direct the central ray perpendicular to the level of the iliac crests.			
6. Center the cassette to the central ray.			
7. Collimate to the abdominal walls laterally and to film size lengthwise; use gonadal shielding, if possible.			
8. Make the exposure during suspended *expiration.*			
9. Obtain both oblique projections or as requested.			

CRITICAL ANATOMY: The kidney furthest from the film will be parallel to the film plane and the ureter nearest the film will be projected away from the spine; overrotation of the patient will project the elevated kidney over the spine.

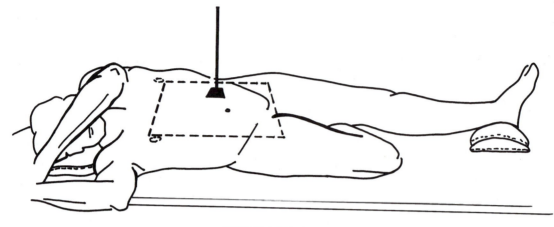

FIGURE 14–3. RPO urinary tract.

NOTES

► AP URINARY BLADDER (UROGRAM OR CYSTOGRAM)

OBJECTIVE: After practice, each student will position a patient for an AP projection of the urinary bladder as performed for an IVP or cystogram.

PATIENT PREP: Remove all clothing except shoes and socks and gown the patient; determine if pre-examination instructions were followed and obtain a pertinent patient history.

FILM: 10 in. × 12 in. crosswise (IVP) or 10 in. × 12 in. lengthwise (cystogram), grid.

TASK ANALYSIS		CORRECTLY PERFORMED?	
MAJOR STEPS	KEY INFORMATION	YES	NO
1. Position the patient supine with the body parallel to the long axis of the table.	The shoulders and pelvis should be adjusted so there is no rotation; sponges may be used for support, if necessary.		
2. Center the midsagittal plane to the midline of the table.	Check body alignment from the head or foot of the table.		
3. Position the patient's arms comfortably at the sides.	Make sure the patient's arms are *not* on the abdomen or tucked under the body.		
4. Direct the central ray 5–20° caudad to the point approximately 2 in. superior to the symphysis pubis.	The central ray should enter at the level of the soft-tissue depression just above the prominent point of the greater trochanter. The degree of central ray angulation should project the symphysis pubis inferior to the bladder and is determined by the amount of lumbar curvature: the greater the curvature, the smaller the central ray angle.		
5. Center the cassette to the central ray.			
6. Collimate to the ASISs crosswise and to the film size lengthwise.			
7. Make the exposure during suspended *expiration*.			

NOTE: *For cystogram studies, lengthwise positioning of the cassette is employed to include the distal ureters and evaluate ureteral reflux.*

CRITICAL ANATOMY: Distal ureters, bladder, and proximal urethra.

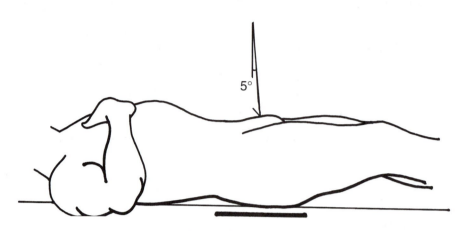

5°

FIGURE 14–4. AP urinary bladder.

NOTES

EVALUATOR SIGNATURE _____ DATE _____

▶ AP OBLIQUE URINARY BLADDER (UROGRAM OR CYSTOGRAM)

OBJECTIVE: After practice, each student will position a patient for AP oblique projections (RPO and LPO) of the urinary bladder.

PATIENT PREP: Remove all clothing except shoes and socks and gown the patient; determine if pre-examination instructions were followed and obtain a pertinent patient history.

FILM: 10 in. × 12 in. lengthwise, grid.

TASK ANALYSIS		CORRECTLY PERFORMED?	
MAJOR STEPS	KEY INFORMATION	YES	NO

1. Assist the patient to the supine position on the table.			
2. Slide the patient approximately 4 in. toward one side of the table.	The patient should still be supine.		
3. Rotate the patient 40–60° toward the opposite side, bringing the patient's independent arm across the chest.	If the patient is moved to the left side of the table, he or she can turn onto the right side and roll backward to a 40–60° oblique position, using a lumbar sponge to support the shoulders and hips. The independent leg should be extended and abducted as much as possible to prevent superimposition over the bladder.		
4. Center the plane passing through the bladder to the midline of the table.	Align the patient to the long axis of the table.		
5. Direct the central ray perpendicular to a point approximately 2 in. superior to the symphysis pubis and 2–3 in. medial to the elevated ASIS.	The central ray should enter at the level of the soft-tissue depression just above the prominent part of the greater trochanter.		
6. Center the cassette to the central ray.	The central ray may also be directed 10° caudad to project the symphysis pubis inferiorly.		
7. Collimate to the bladder area.			
8. Make the exposure during suspended *expiration*.			
9. Obtain both oblique projections or as requested.			

NOTE: *When performed as part of a urogram, the oblique projection may be more shallow. For voiding studies on male patients, the cassette should be centered to the level of the superior border of the pubic symphysis.*

CRITICAL ANATOMY: Posterolateral aspect of the bladder and ureterovesicular junction of the side furthest from the film.

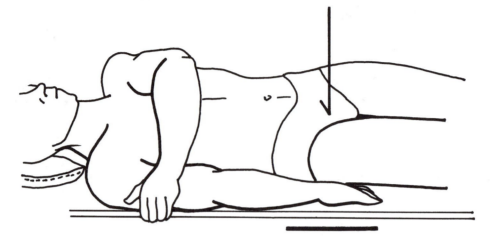

FIGURE 14–5. RPO urinary bladder.

NOTES
....

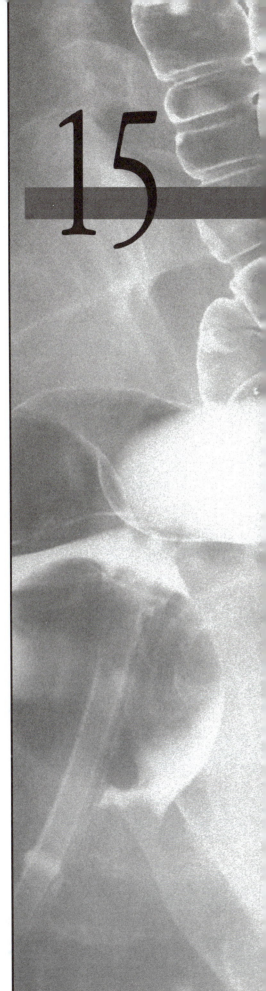

15

DIGESTIVE SYSTEM

► AP ESOPHAGUS

OBJECTIVE: After practice, each student will position a patient for an AP projection of the esophagus.

PATIENT PREP: Remove necklaces and all clothing except shoes and socks and gown the patient; obtain a pertinent patient history.

FILM: 14 in. × 17 in. lengthwise, grid.

TASK ANALYSIS		CORRECTLY PERFORMED?	
MAJOR STEPS	KEY INFORMATION	YES	NO

MAJOR STEPS	KEY INFORMATION
1. Position the patient supine with the body parallel to the long axis of the table.	This projection may be obtained upright; however, the recumbent position allows for more complete filling of the esophagus. The projection may also be obtained with the patient prone.
2. Center the midsagittal plane to the midline of the table.	Check body alignment from the head or foot of the table.
3. Position the patient's arms comfortably at the sides.	
4. Flex the knees and support them with sandbags, sponges, or pillows.	This eases the stress on the patient's back and makes the position more comfortable.
5. Position the cassette so the upper edge is 2 to 3 in. above the top of the shoulders.	
6. Direct the central ray perpendicular to the midpoint of the cassette.	The central ray should enter at the level of T5–6, about 1 in. below the sternal angle.
7. Collimate to an 8-in. field size crosswise and to the film lengthwise; use gonadal shielding.	
8. Instruct the patient to take 1 to 3 spoonfuls or several drinks of thick barium through a straw. The final spoonful or drink should be held in the mouth until instructed to swallow.	The exposure may also be made as the patient is continuously swallowing barium while drinking through a straw.
9. Instruct the patient to exhale, then swallow the barium before taking in another breath.	
10. Make the exposure immediately after the patient swallows the barium.	Respiration is naturally suspended for approximately 2 seconds after swallowing.

CRITICAL ANATOMY: Barium-filled esophagus from the pharynx through the cardiac antrum to the fundus of the stomach.

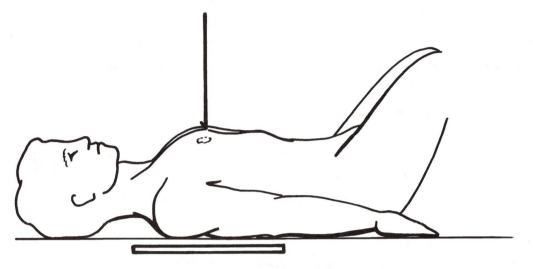

FIGURE 15–1. AP esophagus.

NOTES

► RAO ESOPHAGUS

OBJECTIVE: After practice, each student will position a patient for an RAO projection of the esophagus.

PATIENT PREP: Remove necklaces and all clothing except shoes and socks and gown the patient; obtain a pertinent patient history.

FILM: 14 in. × 17 in. lengthwise, grid.

TASK ANALYSIS		CORRECTLY PERFORMED?	
MAJOR STEPS	KEY INFORMATION	YES	NO
1. Assist the patient to the prone position on the table.	This projection may be obtained upright; however, the recumbent position allows for more complete filling of the esophagus.		
2. Rotate the patient to a 35–40° RAO position.	Thin patients must be rotated more than larger patients to project the esophagus anterior to the spine. The patient may use the left arm and leg for support.		
3. Center the thorax to the midline of the table.			
4. Position the cassette so the upper edge is 2 to 3 in. above the top of the shoulders.			
5. Direct the central ray perpendicular to the midpoint of the cassette.	The central ray should be directed to the level of T5–6, about 1 in. below the level of the sternal angle.		
6. Collimate to an 8-in. field size crosswise and to the film lengthwise; use gonadal shielding.			
7. Instruct the patient to take 1 to 3 spoonfuls or several drinks of thick barium through a straw. The final spoonful or drink should be held in the mouth until instructed to swallow.	The exposure may also be made as the patient is continuously swallowing barium while drinking through a straw.		
8. Instruct the patient to exhale, then swallow the barium before taking in another breath.			
9. Make the exposure immediately after the patient swallows the barium.	Respiration is naturally suspended for approximately 2 seconds after swallowing.		

CRITICAL ANATOMY   Barium-filled esophagus from the pharynx through the cardiac antrum to the fundus of the stomach.

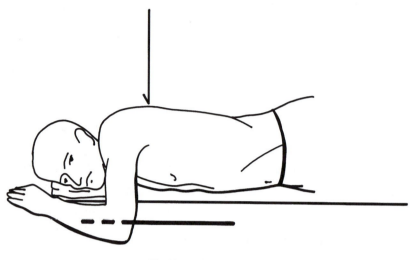

FIGURE 15–2. RAO esophagus.

NOTES
....

► LATERAL ESOPHAGUS

OBJECTIVE: After practice, each student will position a patient for a lateral projection of the esophagus.

PATIENT PREP: Remove necklaces and all clothing except shoes and socks and gown the patient; obtain a pertinent patient history.

FILM: 14 in. × 17 in. lengthwise, grid.

TASK ANALYSIS		CORRECTLY PERFORMED?	
MAJOR STEPS	KEY INFORMATION	YES	NO
1. Assist the patient to the right lateral position on the table.	This projection may be obtained upright; however, the recumbent position allows for more complete filling of the esophagus. The left lateral position may also be used.		
2. Position the arms at a 90° angle with the long axis of the body.	The left arm should be directly over the right arm.		
3. Adjust the patient to a true lateral position.	Flex the knees and hips to a comfortable position.		
4. Center the midcoronal plane to the midline of the table.			
5. Position the cassette so the upper edge is 2 to 3 in. above the top of the shoulders.			
6. Direct the central ray perpendicular to the midpoint of the cassette.	The central ray should be directed to the level of T5–6, about 1 in. below the level of the sternal angle.		
7. Collimate to an 8-in. field size crosswise and to the film lengthwise; use gonadal shielding.			
8. Instruct the patient to take 1 to 3 spoonfuls or several drinks of thick barium through a straw. The final spoonful or drink should be held in the mouth until instructed to swallow.	The exposure may also be made as the patient is continuously swallowing barium while drinking through a straw.		
9. Instruct the patient to exhale, then swallow the barium before taking in another breath.			
10. Make the exposure immediately after the patient swallows the barium.	Respiration is naturally suspended for approximately 2 seconds after swallowing.		

CRITICAL ANATOMY: Barium-filled esophagus from the pharynx through the cardiac antrum to the fundus of the stomach.

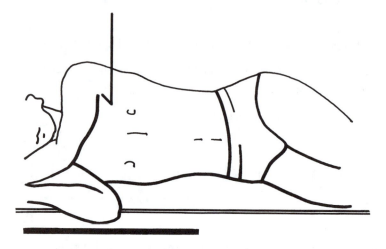

FIGURE 15–3. Lateral esophagus.

NOTES
....

▶ PA STOMACH (UPPER GI)

OBJECTIVE: After practice, each student will position a patient for a PA projection of the stomach and duodenum.

PATIENT PREP: Remove necklaces and all clothing except shoes and socks and gown the patient; obtain a pertinent patient history.

FILM: 10 in. × 12 in., 11 × 14 in., or 14 in. × 17 in. lengthwise, grid.

TASK ANALYSIS		CORRECTLY PERFORMED?	
MAJOR STEPS	KEY INFORMATION	YES	NO
1. Assist the patient to the prone position on the table.	Align the patient to the long axis of the table. This view may also be obtained with the patient supine (AP projection).		
2. Position the patient's arms on the table near the head.	Make sure the patient is lying as flat as possible; the pillow should be positioned only under the head.		

3. Center the midsagittal plane:
  a. To the midline of the table when a 14 in. × 17 in. cassette is used, or
  b. 1 to 2 in. to the right of the table midline for smaller cassettes.
	The sagittal plane 1 to 2 in. to the left of the spine will be centered to the midline of the table. *Note:* Asthenic patients should be positioned so the midsagittal plane corresponds with the midline of the table.		

4. Direct the central ray perpendicular to the level of the duodenal bulb (L-2).	Centering will be slightly below the transpyloric plane and slightly above the inferior margin of the ribs on the average patient. The diaphragm should be included when using 14 in. × 17 in. film.		
5. Center the cassette to the central ray.			
6. Collimate to the abdomen laterally when using a 14 in. × 17 in. cassette and to allow 1/2 in. margins when using smaller cassettes.			
7. Make the exposure during suspended *expiration*.			

NOTE: *Normal centering for hypersthenic patients is to the level of L-1 and to L-3 for asthenic patients. For upright projections, the central ray should be directed 1 to 4 in. lower.*

CRITICAL ANATOMY: Fundus, barium-filled body and pylorus, greater and lesser curvatures, C-loop of the duodenum, and duodenal bulb; when this view is obtained with the patient supine, the barium will fill the fundus.

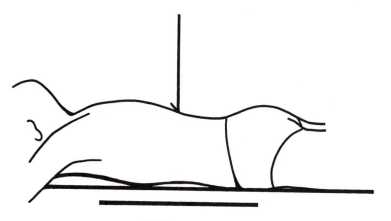

FIGURE 15–4. PA stomach.

NOTES
....

EVALUATOR SIGNATURE _____ DATE _____

▶ RAO STOMACH (UPPER GI)

OBJECTIVE: After practice, each student will position a patient for an RAO projection of the stomach and duodenum.

PATIENT PREP: Remove necklaces and all clothing except shoes and socks and gown the patient; obtain a pertinent patient history.

FILM: 10 in. × 12 in., 11 × 14 in. lengthwise, grid.

TASK ANALYSIS		CORRECTLY PERFORMED?	
MAJOR STEPS	KEY INFORMATION	YES	NO
1. Assist the patient to the RAO position on the table.	The patient should be face down on the table with the right arm near the side and the left arm near the head; the body is rotated so the left side is elevated from the table.		
2. Rotate the patient 40–70°.	To demonstrate the duodenal bulb, hypersthenic patients must be rotated about 70° and asthenic patients about 40°.		
3. Center the longitudinal plane passing midway between the vertebral column and elevated lateral margin of the thorax to the midline of the table.	Align the patient to the long axis of the table.		
4. Direct the central ray perpendicular to the level of the pylorus (L-2) on average patients.	This level is midway between the xiphoid process and the inferior margin of the ribs; centering is slightly higher for hypersthenic patients and slightly lower for asthenic patients.		
5. Center the cassette to the central ray.			
6. Collimate to allow 1/2 in. margins.			
7. Make the exposure during suspended *expiration.*			

NOTE: *The LPO position will give a comparable view, but the contrast medium will fill the fundus.*

CRITICAL ANATOMY: Pyloric canal and duodenal bulb.

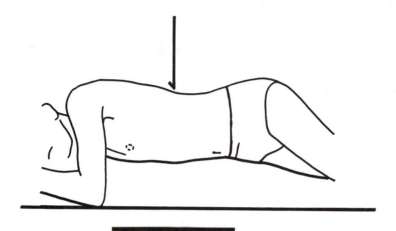

FIGURE 15–5. RAO stomach.

NOTES
....

► LATERAL STOMACH (UPPER GI)

OBJECTIVE: After practice, each student will position a patient for a lateral projection of the stomach and duodenum.

PATIENT PREP: Remove necklaces and all clothing except shoes and socks and gown the patient; obtain a pertinent patient history.

FILM: 10 in. × 12 in. or 11 in. × 14 in. lengthwise, grid.

TASK ANALYSIS		CORRECTLY PERFORMED?	
MAJOR STEPS	KEY INFORMATION	YES	NO
1. Assist the patient to the right lateral position on the table.			
2. Position the arms at a 90° angle with the body.			
3. Center the coronal plane halfway between the midaxillary plane and the anterior abdominal wall to the midline of the table.			
4. Adjust the thorax and pelvis to a true lateral position.	The left arm should be directly over the right arm with the knees flexed slightly for comfort.		
5. Direct the central ray to the level of L-1.	This level is generally halfway between the xiphoid process and the umbilicus.		
6. Center the cassette to the central ray.			
7. Collimate to allow 1/2 in. margins.			
8. Make the exposure during suspended *expiration*.			

NOTE: *Normal centering for hypersthenic patients is to the level of T-12; centering for asthenic patients is to L-2.*

CRITICAL ANATOMY: Pyloric canal and duodenal bulb (especially hypersthenic patients).

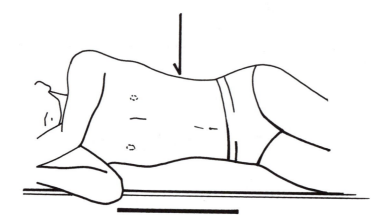

FIGURE 15–6. Right lateral stomach.

NOTES
....

▶ PA & AP SMALL BOWEL

OBJECTIVE: After practice, each student will position a patient for a PA projection of the small intestine.

PATIENT PREP: Remove necklaces and all clothing except shoes and socks and gown the patient; obtain a pertinent patient history.

FILM: 14 in. × 17 in. lengthwise, grid.

TASK ANALYSIS		CORRECTLY PERFORMED?	
MAJOR STEPS	KEY INFORMATION	YES	NO
1. Assist the patient to the prone position on the table.	Align the patient to the long axis of the table. This view may also be obtained with the patient supine (AP projection).		
2. Position the patient's arms on the table near the head.	Make sure the patient is lying as flat as possible; the pillow should be positioned only under the head.		
3. Center the midsagittal plane to the midline of the table.			
4. Direct the central ray perpendicular to: a. The level of the duodenal bulb (L-2), *or* b. The level of the iliac crests.	Obtained for the first film (usually 15 to 30 minutes post-ingestion) to include the diaphragm. Obtained for all subsequent films.		
5. Center the cassette to the central ray.			
6. Collimate to the abdominal walls laterally and to the film size lengthwise.			
7. Make the exposure during suspended *expiration*.			

NOTE: *Films should be appropriately marked with lead markers to indicate the post-ingestion time of the contrast medium.*

CRITICAL ANATOMY: Stomach, duodenum, jejunum, ileum, and proximal large intestine (depending on the post-ingestion time); the radiologist will generally obtain fluoroscopic spot films of the terminal ileum and ileocecal valve.

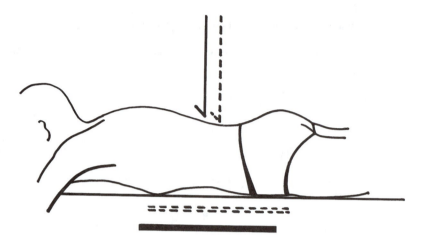

FIGURE 15–7. PA small bowel.

NOTES

▶ AP LARGE INTESTINE (PRELIMINARY, CONTRAST-FILLED & POST-EVACUATION)

OBJECTIVE: After practice, each student will position a patient for an AP projection of the large intestine, with or without contrast.

PATIENT PREP: Remove necklaces and all clothing except shoes and socks and gown the patient; determine if pre-examination instructions were followed and obtain a pertinent patient history. Complete the patient preparation according to department routine.

FILM: 14 in. × 17 in. lengthwise or crosswise (×2) for large patients, grid.

TASK ANALYSIS		CORRECTLY PERFORMED?	
MAJOR STEPS	KEY INFORMATION	YES	NO
1. Assist the patient to the supine position on the table.	The prone position can also be used according to department routine (especially double-contrast studies) or radiologist preference.		
2. Center the midsagittal plane to the midline of the table.	Align the patient to the long axis of the table.		
3. Adjust the patient's body so there is no rotation; the ASISs are equidistant from the table.	Position the patient's arms comfortably at the sides.		
4. Direct the central ray perpendicular to the level of the iliac crests.	For large patients, two 14 in. × 17 in. cassettes should be used crosswise; the first centered to include the symphysis pubis, and the second positioned with at least a 2- to 3-in. overlap of the first.		
5. Center the cassette to the central ray.			
6. Collimate to the abdominal walls laterally and to the film size lengthwise.			
7. Make the exposure during suspended *expiration*.			

CRITICAL ANATOMY: Cecum, ascending colon, transverse colon, and descending colon; when the patient is supine, barium should fill the ascending and descending colon.

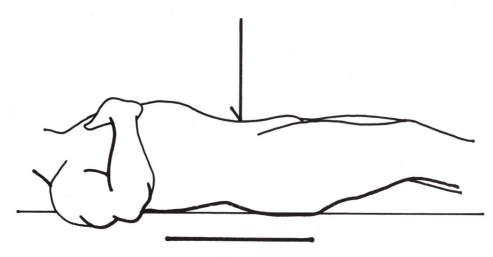

FIGURE 15–8. AP colon.

NOTES
....

▶ PA LARGE INTESTINE (PRELIMINARY, CONTRAST-FILLED & POST-EVACUATION)

OBJECTIVE: After practice, each student will position a patient for a PA projection of the large intestine, with or without contrast.

PATIENT PREP: Remove necklaces and all clothing except shoes and socks and gown the patient; determine if pre-examination instructions were followed and obtain a pertinent patient history. Complete the patient preparation according to department routine.

FILM: 14 in. × 17 in. lengthwise or crosswise (×2) for large patients, grid.

TASK ANALYSIS		CORRECTLY PERFORMED?	
MAJOR STEPS	KEY INFORMATION	YES	NO
1. Assist the patient to the prone position on the table.			
2. Center the midsagittal plane to the midline of the table.	Align the patient to the long axis of the table.		
3. Adjust the patient's shoulders and pelvis so there is no rotation.	Position the patient's arms comfortably near the head; make sure the patient is lying as flat as possible.		
4. Direct the central ray perpendicular to the level of the iliac crests.	For large patients, two 14 in. × 17 in. cassettes should be used crosswise; the first centered to include the symphysis pubis, and the second positioned with at least a 2- to 3-in. overlap of the first.		
5. Center the cassette to the central ray.			
6. Collimate to the abdominal walls crosswise and to the film size lengthwise.			
7. Make the exposure during suspended *expiration.*			

CRITICAL ANATOMY: Cecum, ascending colon, hepatic flexure, transverse colon, splenic flexure, descending colon, sigmoid colon, and rectum; when the patient is prone, barium should fill the transverse colon.

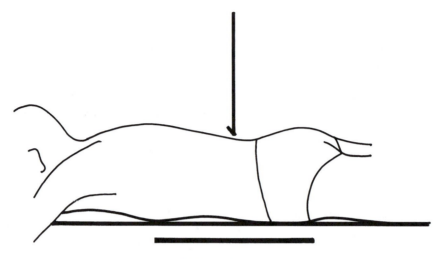

FIGURE 15–9. PA colon.

NOTES
....

▶ AP OBLIQUE LARGE INTESTINE (RPO & LPO)

OBJECTIVE: After practice, each student will position a patient for RPO and LPO projections of the large intestine, with or without contrast.

PATIENT PREP: Remove necklaces and all clothing except shoes and socks and gown the patient; determine if pre-examination instructions were followed and obtain a pertinent patient history. Complete the patient preparation according to department routine.

FILM: 14 in. × 17 in. lengthwise, grid.

TASK ANALYSIS		CORRECTLY PERFORMED?	
MAJOR STEPS	KEY INFORMATION	YES	NO
1. Assist the patient to the supine position on the table.	Posterior oblique, RAO, and LAO projections may also be performed to provide similar views.		
2. Slide the patient approximately 2 to 3 in. toward one side of the table.	Align the patient to the long axis of the table.		
3. Rotate the patient 35–45° toward the opposite side.	If the patient is moved to the left side of the table, he or she can turn toward the right side and be supported by a lumbar sponge positioned behind the shoulders and hips. The entire body should be rotated 35–45°. The patient should bring the left arm across the chest, keeping both hands near the head; the patient can also use the legs for support.		
4. The plane passing through the umbilicus should be centered to the midline of the table.			
5. Direct the central ray perpendicular to the level of the iliac crests.	Check the location of the flexures during fluoroscopy by looking at bony landmarks; adjust centering as necessary. Large patients may require using two 14 in. × 17 in. cassettes crosswise, centering the first film to include the symphysis pubis and the second with a 2- to 3-in. overlap of the first.		
6. Center the cassette to the central ray.			
7. Collimate to the abdominal walls crosswise and to the film size lengthwise.			
8. Make the exposure during suspended *expiration*.			

Continued

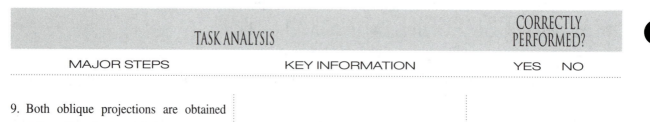

TASK ANALYSIS		CORRECTLY PERFORMED?	
MAJOR STEPS	KEY INFORMATION	YES	NO

9. Both oblique projections are obtained unless otherwise requested.

CRITICAL ANATOMY: *RPO*—Left colonic flexure and descending colon. *LPO*—Right colonic flexure and ascending colon.

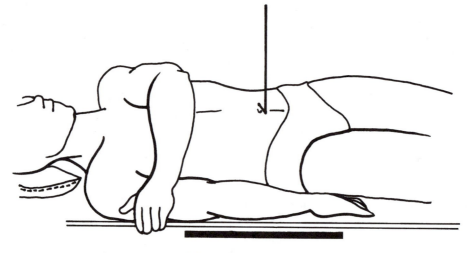

FIGURE 15–10. RPO colon.

NOTES

EVALUATOR SIGNATURE _____ DATE _____

► AP AXIAL RECTOSIGMOID REGION

OBJECTIVE: After practice, each student will position a patient for an AP axial projection of the colon.

PATIENT PREP: Remove necklaces and all clothing except shoes and socks and gown the patient; determine if pre-examination instructions were followed and obtain a pertinent patient history. Complete the patient preparation according to department routine.

FILM: 11 in. × 14 in. or 14 in. × 17 in. lengthwise, grid.

TASK ANALYSIS		CORRECTLY PERFORMED?	
MAJOR STEPS	KEY INFORMATION	YES	NO

MAJOR STEPS	KEY INFORMATION
1. Assist the patient to the supine position on the table.	The shoulders and pelvis should be adjusted so there is no rotation. A similar view may be obtained by positioning the patient prone and directing the central ray caudally.
2. Center the midsagittal plane to the midline of the table.	Align the patient to the long axis of the table.
3. Adjust the patient's body so there is no rotation.	Position the patient's arms on the chest or comfortably at the sides; make sure the patient's arms are *not* positioned on the abdomen or tucked under the body.
4. Direct the central ray 30–45° cephalad to: a. ***11 in. × 14 in. cassette:*** The level of the symphysis pubis. *or* b. ***14 in. × 17 in. cassette:*** A point approximately 2 in. below the level of the ASISs.	
5. Center the cassette to the central ray.	
6. Collimate to film size.	
7. Make the exposure during suspended *expiration.*	

CRITICAL ANATOMY: Rectum and sigmoid colon.

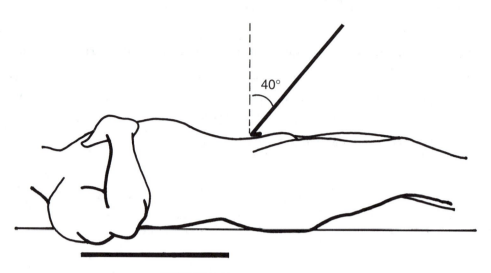

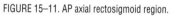

FIGURE 15–11. AP axial rectosigmoid region.

NOTES

EVALUATOR SIGNATURE _____ DATE _____

► LATERAL RECTUM/LARGE INTESTINE (CONTRAST-FILLED & POST-EVACUATION)

OBJECTIVE: After practice, each student will position a patient for a lateral projection of the rectum.

PATIENT PREP: Remove necklaces and all clothing except shoes and socks and gown the patient; determine if pre-examination instructions were followed and obtain a pertinent patient history. Complete the patient preparation according to department routine.

FILM: 11 in. × 14 in., 10 in. × 12 in., or 14 in. × 17 in. lengthwise, grid.

TASK ANALYSIS		CORRECTLY PERFORMED?	
MAJOR STEPS	KEY INFORMATION	YES	NO
1. Assist the patient to the lateral position on the table.	Although the left lateral projection is usually obtained, the patient may also be placed in the right lateral or ventral decubitus (prone) position.		
2. Adjust the thorax and pelvis to a true lateral position.			
3. Position the arms at a 90° angle with the body.			
4. Flex the knees and hips to a comfortable position.	The right arm should be directly over the left arm and the right leg directly over the left leg.		
5. Center the plane 2 in. posterior to the midcoronal plane to the midline of the table.	If a 14 in. × 17 in. cassette is used, the midaxillary plane is centered to the midline of the table.		
6. Direct the central ray perpendicular to the level of the ASIS.	This centering is used for smaller cassettes. If a 14 in. × 17 in. cassette is used, centering is to the level of the iliac crests.		
7. Center the cassette to the central ray.			
8. Collimate to allow 1/2 in. margins.			
9. Make the exposure during suspended *expiration.*			

CRITICAL ANATOMY: Rectum and rectosigmoid area.

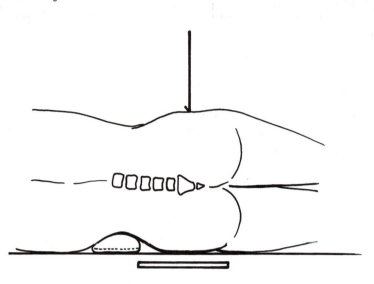

FIGURE 15–12. Lateral rectum.

NOTES

EVALUATOR SIGNATURE _____ DATE _____

▶ LATERAL DECUBITUS LARGE INTESTINE (DOUBLE-CONTRAST STUDIES)

OBJECTIVE: After practice, each student will position a patient for a lateral decubitus projection of the large intestine.

PATIENT PREP: Remove necklaces and all clothing except shoes and socks and gown the patient; determine if pre-examination instructions were followed and obtain a pertinent patient history. Complete the patient preparation according to department routine.

FILM: 14 in. × 17 in. crosswise (lengthwise with the patient).

TASK ANALYSIS		CORRECTLY PERFORMED?	
MAJOR STEPS	KEY INFORMATION	YES	NO
1. Assist the patient to the lateral position on the table.	Both right and left lateral decubitus, AP or PA, projections are usually obtained. Radiolucent supports may be needed to position the patient in the middle of the film. The patient may also be positioned on a stretcher in front of a vertical grid device.		
2. Adjust the thorax and pelvis to a true lateral position.	Rotation can easily be checked by standing at the head or foot of the table.		
3. Keeping the patient lateral, extend the arms upward so the elbows are near the head.			
4. Flex the knees and hips to a comfortable position.	The right arm should be directly over the left arm and the right leg directly over the left leg.		
5. A vertically supported grid cassette should be positioned so it is centered to the level of the iliac crests.	If the patient is on a stretcher, the stretcher should be moved so the iliac crests are centered to the midline of the vertical grid device.		
6. Direct the central ray horizontally to the middle of the grid cassette.	If a vertical grid device is used, the central ray is directed horizontally to the midsagittal plane of the patient; center the cassette to the central ray.		
7. Collimate to the abdominal walls crosswise and to the film size lengthwise.			
8. Make the exposure during suspended *expiration*.			

CRITICAL ANATOMY: *Right lateral decubitus*—Descending colon and left colonic flexure. *Left lateral decubitus*—Ascending colon and right colonic flexure.

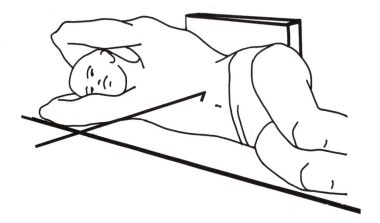

FIGURE 15–13. Right lateral decubitus colon.

NOTES
....

BILIARY SYSTEM

16

► PA GALLBLADDER (CHOLECYSTOGRAM)

OBJECTIVE: After practice, each student will position a patient for a PA scout and localized projections of the abdomen for demonstration of the gallbladder (cholecystogram).

PATIENT PREP: Remove all clothing except shoes and socks and gown the patient; determine if pre-examination instructions were followed and obtain a pertinent patient history.

FILM: 14 in. × 17 in. or 10 in. × 12 in. lengthwise, grid.

TASK ANALYSIS		CORRECTLY PERFORMED?	
MAJOR STEPS	KEY INFORMATION	YES	NO
1. Assist the patient to the prone position on the table with a pillow supporting the head.	This projection may also be obtained with the patient upright to demonstrate stratification of stones.		
2. *Abdominal scout using a 14 in. × 17 in. cassette:*			
a. Center the midsagittal plane to the midline of the table.	The sagittal plane 2 to 3 in. (depending on patient size) to the right of the spine may also be centered to the table. Align the patient to the long axis of the table.		
b. Direct the central ray perpendicular to the level of the iliac crests.	Tall patients may require centering as much as 2 to 3 in. above the iliac crests.		
c. Center the cassette to the central ray.			
d. Collimate to the abdomen laterally and to the film size lengthwise; use gonadal shielding, if possible.			
e. Make the exposure during suspended *expiration.*			
3. *Localized view using a 10 in. × 12 in. cassette:*			
a. Center the sagittal plane midway between the spine and lateral margin of the ribs to the midline of the table.	Align the patient to the long axis of the table.		
b. Direct the central ray perpendicular to the level of the inferior margin of the ribs.			
c. Center the cassette to the central ray.			
d. Collimate to allow at least 1/2-in. margins; use gonadal shielding.			
e. Make the exposure during suspended *expiration.*			

NOTE: *The position of the gallbladder varies with body habitus: higher, more lateral and transverse in hypersthenic patients; lower, closer to the spine, and vertical in asthenic patients. The radiographer must evaluate the patient's body habitus before centering.*

CRITICAL ANATOMY: Fundus, body, and neck of the gallbladder.

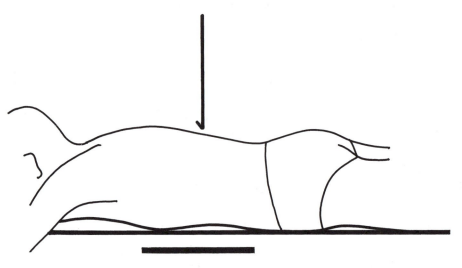

FIGURE 16–1. PA gallbladder.

NOTES
....

► LAO GALLBLADDER (CHOLECYSTOGRAM)

OBJECTIVE: After practice, each student will position a patient for an LAO projection of the gallbladder (cholecystogram).

PATIENT PREP: Remove all clothing except shoes and socks and gown the patient; determine if pre-examination instructions were followed and obtain a pertinent patient history.

FILM: 8 in. × 10 in. or 10 in. × 12 in. lengthwise, or 9 in. × 9 in., grid.

TASK ANALYSIS		CORRECTLY PERFORMED?	
MAJOR STEPS	KEY INFORMATION	YES	NO
1. Assist the patient to the prone position on the table with a pillow supporting the head.	The patient should be aligned to the long axis of the table; this projection may also be obtained with the patient upright to demonstrate stratification of stones.		
2. Rotate the patient to a 15–40° LAO position.	The amount of rotation is determined by the body habitus: very thin patients must be rotated more than hypersthenic patients in order to separate the gallbladder from the spine. The patient should use the right arm and leg for support.		
3. Center the sagittal plane midway between the lateral margin of the ribs and the spine to the midline of the table.			
4. Direct the central ray perpendicular to the level of the last rib.	Exact centering is determined by the patient's body habitus: lower for thin patients and higher for larger patients.		
5. Center the cassette to the central ray.			
6. Collimate to allow at least 1/2-in. margins; use gonadal shielding.			
7. Make the exposure during suspended *expiration*.			

NOTE: *Patients who cannot lie on their abdomen or who are having a T-tube cholangiogram performed should be placed in the RPO position.*

CRITICAL ANATOMY: Fundus, body, and neck of the gallbladder.

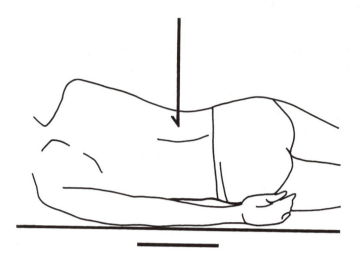

FIGURE 16–2. LAO gallbladder.

NOTES

EVALUATOR SIGNATURE _____ DATE _____

▶ RIGHT LATERAL DECUBITUS GALLBLADDER (CHOLECYSTOGRAM)

OBJECTIVE: After practice, each student will position a patient for a right lateral decubitus projection of the gallbladder (cholecystogram).

PATIENT PREP: Remove all clothing except shoes and socks and gown the patient; determine if pre-examination instructions were followed and obtain a pertinent patient history.

FILM: 8 in. × 10 in. or 10 in. × 12 in. lengthwise, or 9 in. × 9 in., grid.

TASK ANALYSIS		CORRECTLY PERFORMED?	
MAJOR STEPS	KEY INFORMATION	YES	NO
1. Turn the radiographic table to the 90° upright position.	A wall unit or portable grid may also be used.		
2. Assist the patient to the right lateral decubitus position on a stretcher.	The right lateral decubitus is performed so the gallbladder falls away from the spine.		
3. Extend the patient's arms above the head, keeping the left arm directly over the right arm.			
4. Position the stretcher against the upright table or grid device so the patient is facing the table.	The patient's abdomen should be as close to the table as possible. *Lock the stretcher wheels.* **Note:** This projection can also be obtained with the patient facing away from the vertical grid device (AP projection).		
5. Adjust the pelvis and thorax to a true lateral position.	Check to be sure lines passing through the hips and shoulders are perpendicular to the floor or table.		
6. Position the stretcher so the level of the bottom of the last rib corresponds with the midline of the grid device.	For the average patient, the transverse plane 2 to 3 in. above the iliac crests is centered to the midline of the grid. If the patient is on the table and a vertical grid cassette is used, the cassette, rather than the patient, can be moved. Exact positioning of the gallbladder varies and is dependent on the patient's body habitus. The PA radiograph should be used to assist in centering.		
7. Direct the central ray horizontally to the center of the table through the plane passing halfway between the lateral margin of the ribs and the spine.			
8. Center the cassette to the central ray.			

Continued

TASK ANALYSIS		CORRECTLY PERFORMED?	
MAJOR STEPS	KEY INFORMATION	YES	NO

9. Collimate to allow at least 1/2-in. margins on all sides.

10. Make the exposure during suspended *expiration.*

NOTE: *This projection allows any calculi to layer within the gallbladder. Upright projections may be substituted for this projection.*

CRITICAL ANATOMY: Fundus, body, and neck of the gallbladder.

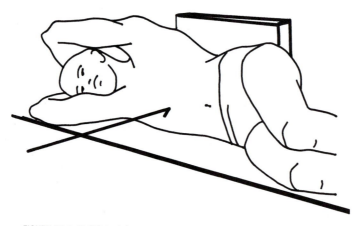

FIGURE 16–3. Right lateral decubitus gallbladder, AP projection, using a portable grid.

NOTES

EVALUATOR SIGNATURE _____ DATE _____

BIBLIOGRAPHY

Ballinger PW. *Merrill's Atlas of Radiographic Positions and Radiologic Procedures.* 8th ed., Vol. 1–3. St. Louis: Mosby–Year Book; 1995.

Bontrager KL. *Textbook of Radiographic Positioning and Related Anatomy.* 3rd ed. St. Louis: Mosby–Year Book; 1993.

Cornuelle AG, Gronefeld DH. *Radiographic Anatomy & Positioning: An Integrated Approach.* Stamford, Conn.: Appleton & Lange; 1998.

Ehrlich RA, McCloskey ED. *Patient Care in Radiography.* 4th ed. St. Louis: Mosby–Year Book; 1993.

McQuillen-Martensen K. *Radiographic Critique.* Philadelphia: W.B. Saunders Company; 1996.